10-20-30 training: Little effort to lose fat, improve health and performance –

also effective to handle diabetes, hypertension and asthma

Jens Bangsbo

10-20-30 training: Little effort to lose fat, improve health and performance – also effective to handle diabetes, hypertension and asthma

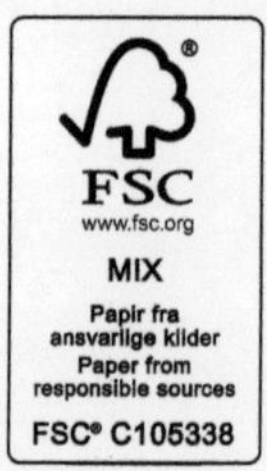

Publisher: BoD – Books on Demand, Hellerup, Denmark

Print: BoD – Books on Demand, Norderstedt, Germany

ISBN: 978-87-4305-799-4

About the author

Jens Bangsbo is Professor at the Department for Sports and Nutrition, University of Copenhagen, Denmark, which is the number one Sport Science department in the world. He has written over 350 scientific articles and more than 25 books about training based on his research and scientific knowledge. He is considered one of the world's leading sports scientists and renowned for his ability to transfer science to practice. He is the inventor of the 10-20-30 training method and has conducted a high number of scientific studies examining the effect of the 10-20-30 training on untrained, trained, well-trained as well as patient groups, such as hypertensive, diabetes and asthma patients. He is former professional soccer player, FIFA instructor, UEFA pro-license and top-class soccer coach being assistant coach at several successful football teams such as Juventus FC, Italy, the Danish national team and Atalanta FC, Italy for the past five years.

A Danish runners now aged 67 years, who has been running for nearly thirty years:

"For me, interval training was associated with something deadly, servile and something that hurt. You know, the classic excuses and pretenses. That's why I had always avoided it in my running training". "By chance, I heard about the 10-20-30 training. I thought that the program was clear and gave it a try. After making 10-20-30 part of my training, I improved his marathon time by 40 minutes even after a three-year break from marathon running".

"Common logic says that a man of my age should just get slower and slower because of biology. Therefore, there is only one explanation for my improved result: the use of interval training with 10-20-30. There is simply no other justification".

"I runs three times a week, and do 10-20-30 twice a week".

 "I am surprised that it is over so quickly. The 10-20-30 training only takes about half an hour. And the sprints are almost over before they really burn. Still, I can feel that I have really used my body. I'm hooked!".

Foreword

At our work at the Department of Sport and Nutrition at the University of Copenhagen, ranked number one university in the world within sport four years in a row, we have made many attempts to find the most effective form of training to improve performance and health. We conducted a series of studies in which experienced runners performed training with 30-second intervals at near maximum speed followed by some minutes breaks. It turned out that this form of training was extremely effective, and that the runners improved performance over both short and long distances, despite the fact that the amount of training was significantly reduced.

However, the 30 seconds of intense exercise is though. If you only ask for 10 seconds, it is much easier, and you almost feel like you are done before you start. This is how the 10-20-30 training concept came about. It turned out that training not only improved performance, but also - to our great surprise - health. We have also found, that it is the most effective and inspiring training for various patients groups, such as hypertensive, diabetes and asthma patients. It is now a commonly used training method and with this book, I will like to provide you with clear guidelines for how to conduct the training. You can easily and safely get started with the 10-20-30 training, whether you want to run or cycle.

Have a nice 10-20-30 training.

Jens Bangsbo

Content

Diabetes patients

- 10-20-30 training of diabetes patients
- Effect of 10-20-30 training on long-term blood glucose of diabetes patients
- Effect of 10-20-30 training on body composition of diabetes patients
- Effect of 10-20-30 training on maximum oxygen uptake and performance of diabetes patients
- Perspectives for diabetes patients
- 10-20-30 training programme for diabetes patients

Hypertensive

- 10-20-30 training of hypertensive
- Effect of 10-20-30 training on blood pressure for hypertensive
- Effect of 10-20-30 training on maximum oxygen uptake and performance of hypertensive
- Perspectives of 10-20-30 training for hypertensive
- 10-20-30 training programme for hypertensive

Asthma patients

- 10-20-30 training of asthma patients
- Effect of 10-20-30 training and diet on asthma control and quality of life for asthma patients
- Effect of 10-20-30 training and diet on body composition in asthma patients
- Effect of 10-20-30 training and diet on maximum oxygen uptake and performance of asthma patients
- Perspectives of 10-20-30 training for asthma patients
- 10-20-30 training programme for asthma patients

Introduction

In the first scientific study with the 10-20-30 training, recreational runners did not only improve their performance, despite a 50%-reduction in training volume, they also surprisingly decreased their blood pressure and got a better blood fat profile. Since then a number of studies with the 10-20-30 training have been carried out also with previous sedentary people confirming that the training is very effective. Actually in a brand new study it was shown that the improvements with the 10-20-30 training where the participant only did 80% of maximal effort during the 10-second intervals, were as great as when the 10-second intervals were done maximally. In recent years, the 10-20-30 method has also been applied to various patient groups, such as hypertensive, diabetes and asthma patients. The results have been amazing. Despite the limited training time and volume, they improved health significantly and reduced the problems with the disease. Importantly, the patients did not face any problems in conducting the training and continued the training after the projects were completed. The training is performed in a short time and is very time efficient, which makes it feasible even for busy people. The training can be done running or cycling individually or in groups.

This book describes how to conduct the 10-20-30 training and the many positive effects of the training. Also how you can measure your progress. It provides a series of customized programmes, whether you are beginner, have many years of training experience or are hypertensive, have diabetes or asthma. The 10-20-30 training is simple to conduct whether it is home, outside, in a fitness center or in a hospital setting, and all can improve.

What is 10-20-30 training?

10-20-30 training is a form of training, where exercise intensity, i.e. running speed or loading/pedaling frequency on a bike, is often changed. It is performed in the order 30-20-10. Low intensity for 30 seconds, followed by 20 seconds at a moderate pace, and then 10 seconds with high intensity. This takes a minute and is repeated five times. Then a 1-4-minute break. Such 5-minute periods are performed 1-4 times in a training session.

Figure 1 shows an example of the running speed (km per hour) measured with GPS during a 10-20-30 training for a runner, who conducted two 5-minute periods. His top speed was 18 km per hour. As it turns out, the speed of the last sprint was significantly lower as he had become tired.

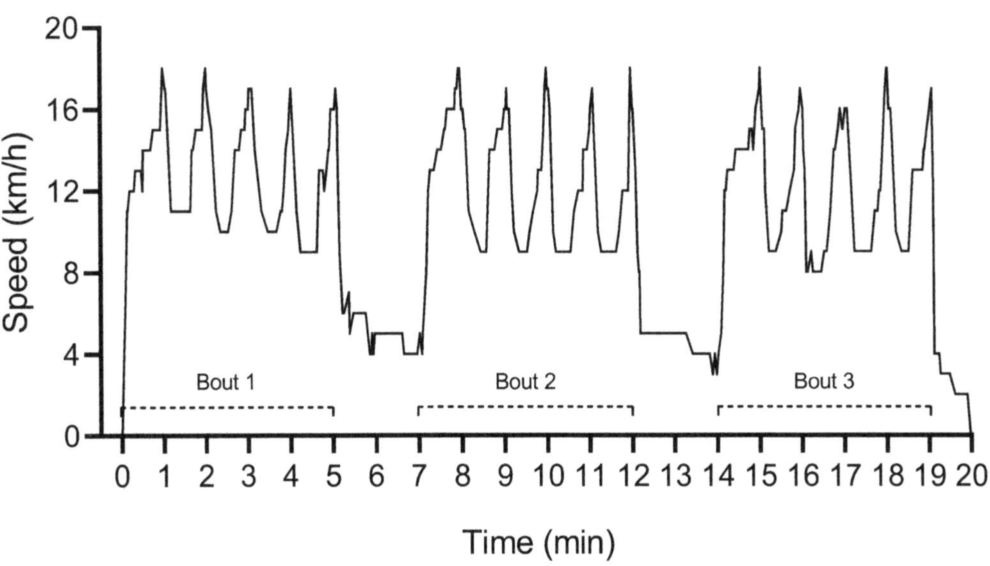

Figure 1. Running speed during 10-20-30 training for a runner.

The cycle training can be performed on a bike at home or at a fitness center. Figure 2B shows an example of the loading of a person conducting 10-20-30 training on a cycle. The cycle 10-20-30 training can also be conducted outside, you just need to find a route without obstacles, such as traffic lights. A possibility is to select a route with a hill. Then, for the 10 seconds you are biking up the hill, turning and relaxing when going down the hill and further on a flat part, then turning around after 30 seconds and then the 20 seconds with moderate speed at the flat part before a new 10-second interval uphill.

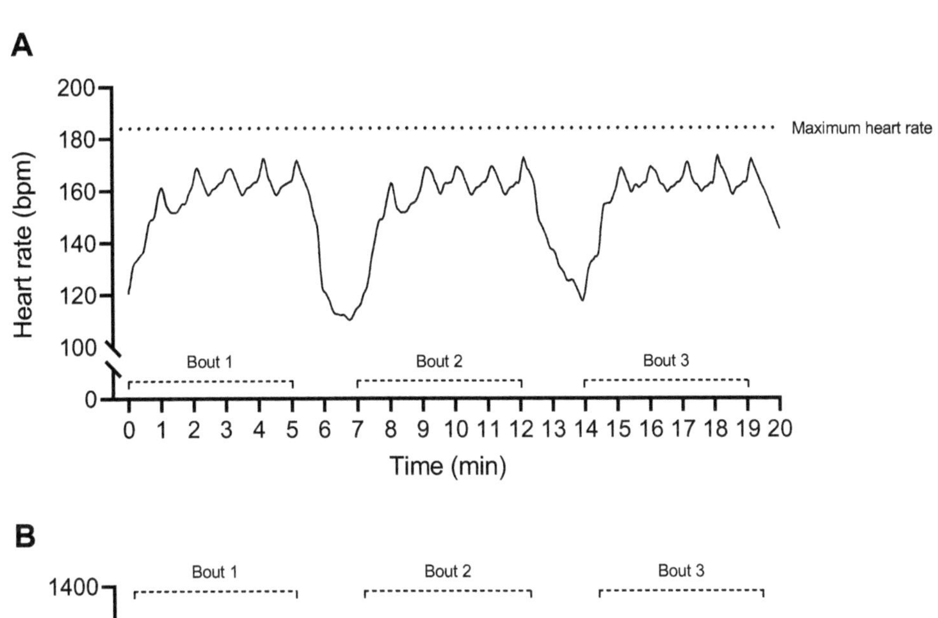

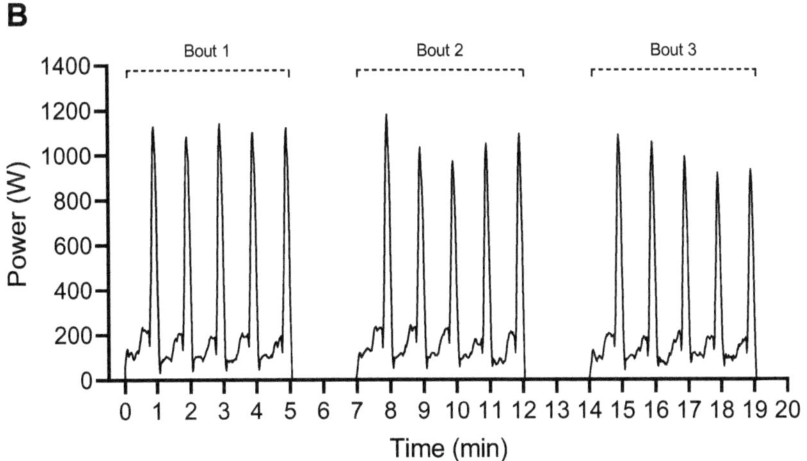

Figure 2. Heart rate (A) and power output (B) during a 10-20-30 cycle training session.

To get started

The first time you conduct 10-20-30 training start slowly. You may walk or cycle without load during the 30 seconds. Do not perform maximally during the final 10 seconds, but rather increase the intensity moderately. Perform one or two five-minute blocks and have a longer break than the suggested 2 minutes between repetitions. If you are running, it is an advantage, if you the first times are running back and forth on the same route. That is, after the first round with 30 seconds of slow running, 20 seconds of normal running and 10 seconds faster running, turn around and start with a new round of 30 seconds slow running, 20 seconds of normal running and 10 seconds faster run, the opposite way. This allows you to see you running distance in each 1-minute period, and you get a sense of what speeds that are optimal for you. Do not be alarmed, if you stay breathless by the workout. Even though the 10-second high intensity does not sound of much, it will feel strenuous in the beginning, but you will quickly get used to it. It is preferable to conduct the training with somebody else, so you can share your experiences and, in time, you may push each other during training.

When you have get used to the 10-20-30 training, you should increase the intensity during the 10-second periods. Do not feel though completely exhausted after the 10 seconds, and if you have not recovered before the next 10-second period, you need to reduce the intensity during the 20 seconds of moderate intensity.

As you become more experienced, you can increase the number of 5-minute periods to three and later four times in a training session (see programs later).

Warm-up

Training should always be started with a 5-minute warm-up period. The first 2 minutes it may be jogging or cycling without loading, then, the next 3 minutes with a slightly higher running speed or loading on the bike.

Keep track of time

With the specially developed 10-20-30 app (Løb -10-20-30 – Apps i Google Play) you get a tool to keep track of when you need to change tempo. The app can be set to the desired number of intervals, and then it controls with sound or vibration, when is the time to switch between the different intensities. Alternatively, you may just use a watch.

"It's surprisingly easy to hit the right times. I count to eight at my own slow pace when I sprints and it fits just right. In the beginning, I tended to ask for a little too long, but now I have modified". Man aged 46 years.

How should I fell during the 10-20-30 training?

After getting used to the 10-20-30 training, you should feel out of breath at the end of each 5-minute interval. Here the following 2-4-minute recovery break should feel like a welcome break. You can use the scale in Table 1 to get an idea of how much you must exert yourself. Before the 10-second period, that is, after the 20 seconds at moderate intensity, you have to feel the load, like somehow strenuous, so around 12-14 on the scale. After the 10-second period, you may reach 17-18, but not maximum strain (19-20). After the 30-second period, you must be around 10-11.

Table 1. Experienced effort

Scale	Perceived effort
6	No effort
7	Very very easy
8	
9	Very easy
10	
11	Pretty easy
12	
13	Something strenuous
14	
15	Tiring
16	
17	Very strenuous
18	
19	Very very strenuous
20	Maximum effort

Measuring heart rate during 10-20-30 training

Heart rate provides a good indication of your loading during the 10-20-30 training. If you have a heart rate monitor, it is obvious to use that when doing 10-20-30 training. A heart rate monitor measures how often your heart beats per minute, and that number is called the heart rate.

Typically, a heart rate monitor consists of a watch you have on your wrist, and a belt placed around the chest. The belt records when the heart beats and transmits the number to the clock, where the number is shown on the display. In order to get the optimal outcome of the heart rate measurements, it is useful to know your maximum heart rate. Previously, as a rule of thumb the maximum heart rate was suggested to be 220 (beats per minute) minus the age, i.e. 180 beats per minute for a person 40 years of age, but that rule is not valid, as there is a large range in the maximum heart rate among people of the same age. Therefore, it is best, but also the hardest, that you make a test of the maximum heart rate (see below). However, it you are beginner or patients you should not do the test until you have trained a few months.

Figure 3 shows the heart rate during 10-20-30 running training. It is clear that the heart rate is significant higher during 10-20-30 training than during normal constant speed run, which for the runner was around 165 beats per minute.

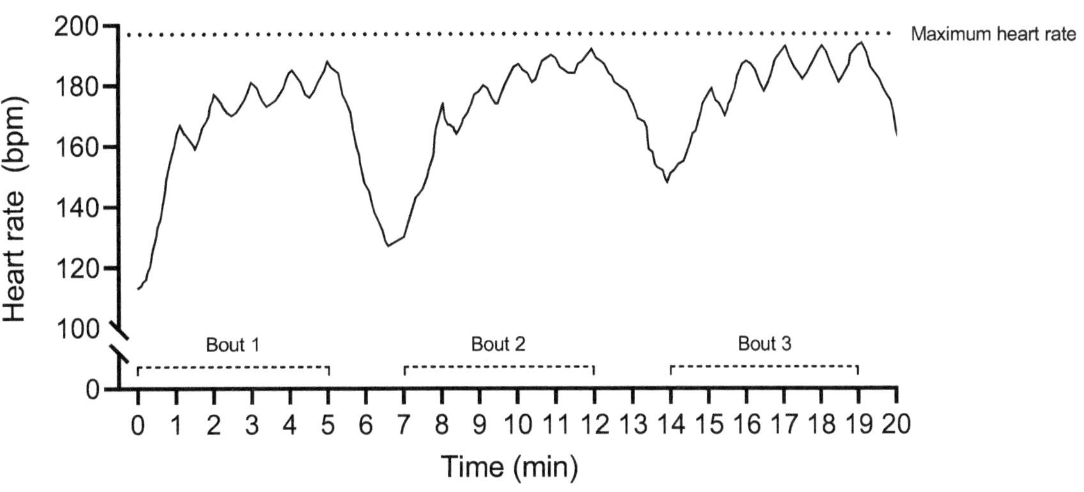

Figure 3. Heart rate during 10-20-30 running training.

Measure heart rate with a finger

You do not need a heart rate monitor to measure your heart rate. You can also measure it by putting a finger on the wrist or on the side of the throat. You should fell the puls "pounding". Once you find the pulse, use a clock and count the number of heart beats for 15 seconds. Multiply the number by 4, as the heart rate is expressed as number of beats per minute. Thus, if you count 35 beats in 15 seconds, your heart rate is 140 beats per minute (35 * 4 = 140 beats per minute). If you count for 30 seconds, you should multiply with 2. Just after the 5-minute intervals during the 10-20-30 training, however, you should not count for longer than 15 seconds, as the heart rate drops rapidly after you stop exercising

When you are experienced with the 10-20-30 training the heart rate after each 5-minute period should preferably be over 85% of your maximum heart rate, e.g. for a person with a maximum heart rate of 190 beats per minute, the heart rate should be above 161 beats per minute (85 percent of 190). In Table 2 you can see the desired heart rate when finishing a 5-minute period dependent of your maximum heart rate. If your heart rate is lower, you may increase the intensity in the 20-second periods.

Table 2. The table shows the lowest heart rate you should have at the end of each 5-minute period depending on your maximum heart rate, when you get experienced with the 10-20-30 training.

Table 2. The table shows the lowest heart rate you should have at the end of each 5-minute period depending on your maximum heart rate, when you get experienced with the 10-20-30 training.

Maximum heart rate (beats per minute)	10-20-30 training heart rate (beats per minute)
160	136
165	140
170	145
175	149
180	153
185	157
190	162
195	166
200	170
205	174
210	179

"The 10-20-30 training is more fun than running a constant speed. Maybe because you are so focused. And then it's more rapidly done". Women 28 years.

How to determine maximum heart rate

The maximum heart rate can be determined by doing gradually increasing intensity running or cycling. Start with moderate speed in 5 minutes, and then increase the intensity every 30 seconds until you are not able to keep the intensity anymore. Immediately after, measure the heart rate or read the heart rate on the heart rate monitor. It is strenuous to determine the maximum heart rate, since your body must be maximally loaded. So prepare to be exhausted. In turn, you only need to do the maximum heart rate test once a year as the maximum heart rate does not depend on changes in your fitness level, but only on age. Your maximum heart rate drops by an average of one beat per minute per year.

Heart rate monitors

Heart rate monitors (see photo) are available in many different variants. Heart rate watches can also work like stop watches and many of the more advanced ones have also GPS built in, so you can measure how far and how fast you run.

The heart rate monitor can also provide information about how many calories you are burning. The measurements are, however, far from accurate.

The most important of the heart rate function is to show your heart rate, thus, how many beat your heart beats per minute.

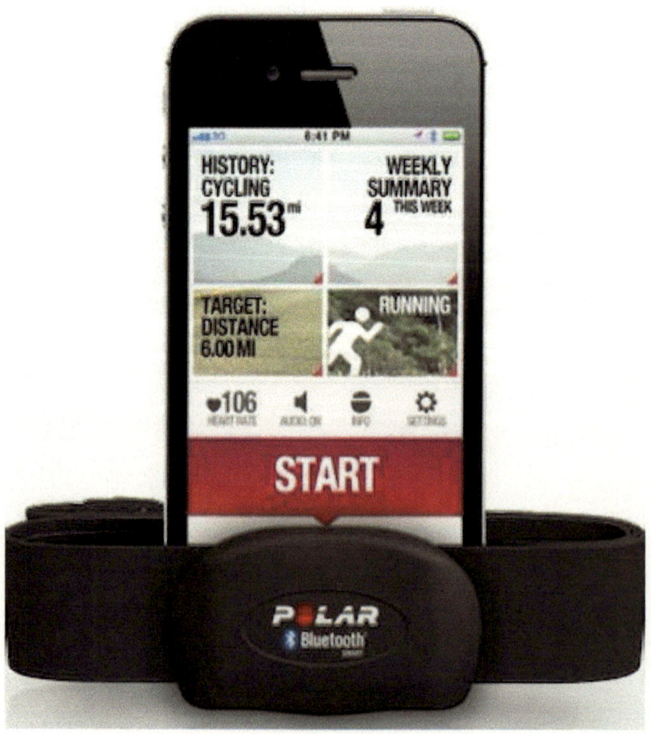

10-20-30 training feels easier

The good thing about the very intense work during 10-20-30 training is that it only lasts 10 seconds, and that you immediately can see an end of it. Many like this type of training and fell that after the active recovery they are well prepared for the next intense work. You got like camouflaged the hard form of training, which elevates the quality of the high intense work.

In a study comparing the effect of 10-20-30 training with another type of interval training, i.e. 30 seconds of running followed by 30 seconds of rest, the participants reported that the 10-20-30 training was much less demanding than the 30-30 training (scale 15 vs. 17 – see Table 1) and also that the perceived exertion decreased dramatically (to 13) during 8 weeks of 10-20-30 training. It can also be mentioned, that despite a significant less relative effort and less volume of training in the 10-20-30 compared to the 30-30 training group (11.6 vs. 15.1 km), the improvements in maximum oxygen uptake and performance were the same in the two groups.

"The sprints are almost over at the moment, I got up to speed. Therefore it feels much easier". Man 37 years.

10-20-30 training brings you together

The runners who trained together experienced that it was a nice social form of training. Runners with very different levels were running together. They got apart during the 10-second sprints, but they could quickly find their way together again during the recovery periods. In addition, they had the time to talk in the breaks between the 5-minute blocks in the 10-20-30 training.

"I had my daughter at 5 years and her friend with me, and I was running in a park. They played while I was running". Mother aged 33 years

What if I get injured?

The risk of getting injured with the 10-20-30 training doing running is limited, and almost no one has been injured during cycle training. Anyway, if you get injured, it is important that you react. Typical injuries in running can be a sprained ankle, if you wiggle, or a sprain in the back of the thigh muscles. In this case, you must stop immediately and quickly starting treatment according to the RICE principle, which stands for R = Rest, I = Ice, C = Compression and E = elevation.

That is, you should not load the foot or leg (Rest). Put ice on the damaged place (Ice). It can be ice cubes in a plastic bag or a bag of frozen peas. Put a towel in between, so you do not get frostbites on your skin. Keep the ice on for about half an hour. Repeat this 3-4 times during the first day. Put tape or elastic band (Compression) around the place and keep that on for a few hours. Then you repeat it the next two days. In the first few hours after the injury is also appropriate having the leg raised high (Elevation), and every time in the next 24 hours when you have an opportunity. For example, put your leg up when you watch television. The RICE principle is used to limit bleeding in the damaged tissues, as it otherwise will delay the healing process and increase the recovery time, and thus, the time until you can get started again.

For major injuries, you should seek a doctor or emergency room to get a professional assessment of the extent of the injury. For minor damage, such as overload, inflammation and general tenderness, you need to reduce the training for a period until you can train again without pain.

Need to recover

If you are tired or do not feel like doing a normal 10-20-30-training session, you may take a day off. Alternatively, you complete an active recovery session that is to perform the 10-20-30 training as 30 seconds walking/no load when cycling, 20 seconds jogging/low load when cycling and 10 seconds of normal running speed/moderate loading when cycling. This is done without warming-up for 15-20 minutes without breaks.

Synopsis – how to do 10-20-30 training

The 10-20-30 training is easy to do. Start with moderate speed or loadings, and then gradually increase as you get used to the training. Do not get worried, that you do not do enough; you will experience the benefits even with a limited effort.

Back in January, I read the abstract for the 10-20-30 training model and started doing those runs. I am a 54 yr old woman who runs a 30 minute 5k. Once a week I run with a 26 yr old young man who is much faster. We switched over to 10-20-30 runs for our weekly runs about 5 weeks ago. We are both totally hooked. Since I am so much slower, he keeps pace with me on warm-ups, recovery and 30 sec intervals. For 20 sec and 10 sec intervals, he runs ahead and then circles back to wherever I am at. We both get a good work out and are completely enjoying our runs. One aspect of the training that I don't remember seeing mentioned in all of the reporting is that this training is consistently giving us both a runner's high. It's so pronounced we both started talking about it on our last run. This makes a lot of sense to me. The 10 sec interval creates enough stress to trigger the endorphins and the recovery periods give enough rest to prevent over-tiring. I just wanted to complement the team that worked on this. It's really rare to find a training program that works so wonderfully. As a slow runner, it's great for me to know that my running partner is going to get a good workout and we are both going to walk away feeling good. I'm also grateful that this work benefits the average runner. A lot of sports research is aimed at olympic runners. This research is something anyone out there can adopt. It is just a really nice piece of work. Women, USA

Effect of 10-20-30 training

This chapter describes the effects of 10-20-30 training based on a number of scientific studies. In one of the studies male and female recreational runners aged between 22-44 years with more than two years of running experience participated. Their normally were running 2-4 times a week with a total distance of approximately 30 km. Running speed was constant and about 11.5 km per hour corresponding to 5½ minutes per km. For seven weeks, the participants completed 10-20-30 training 3 times per week consisting of 3 x 5 minutes for the first 4 weeks, and 4 x 5 minutes the last 3 weeks. The warm up for each session was a 1.2-km run at a moderate pace. The total volume was 13 km in the first weeks and 16 km in the following weeks. Thus, on average the distance was about half the normal distance. Both before and after the 7 weeks the participants underwent series of tests and physical measurements.

10-20-30 training does increase maximum oxygen uptake

The maximum oxygen uptake expressed how well a person is to transport and utilize oxygen in the body, and is often presented as milliliters (ml) oxygen per minute per kilo of body weight. The person running on a treadmill or cycling with a mask, so the exhaled air continuously is transferred for analysis, which makes is possible to measure oxygen uptake. To determine the maximum oxygen uptake, the running speed or the loading on the cycle is progressively increased until the person cannot maintain the speed or the pedal frequency. Untrained woman and men typically have maximum oxygen uptake values around 30-35 and 35-40 ml per minute per kg, respectively, while top-class female and male runners and cyclists have values of about 80 and 90 ml per minute kg, respectively.

The group of trained runners described above had on average maximum oxygen uptake of 52 milliliters per minute per kg before the 10-20-30 training and improved their maximum oxygen uptake by 4% (see Figure 4) after changing to the 10-20-30 training for seven weeks, despite the marked reduction in total running distance. Another group of recreational runners aged 33 years, with a total distance of 15 km per week, also increased maximum oxygen uptake (by 10%) when conducting 3-4 5-minute blocks of 10-20-30 training for eight weeks (see Figure 4). Likewise, a group of untrained men aged 55-65 years doing 10-20-30 cycle training twice a week for six weeks had an increase in maximum oxygen uptake (see Figure 4).

Interestingly when two group of runners performing 10-20-30 training for 6 weeks, where one group did only 80% of maximal effort during the 10-second intervals, no difference in the improvement of maximum oxygen uptake was observed (see Figure 5). This means that even less than maximal effort in the 10-second periods can have the same effect as doing maximally.

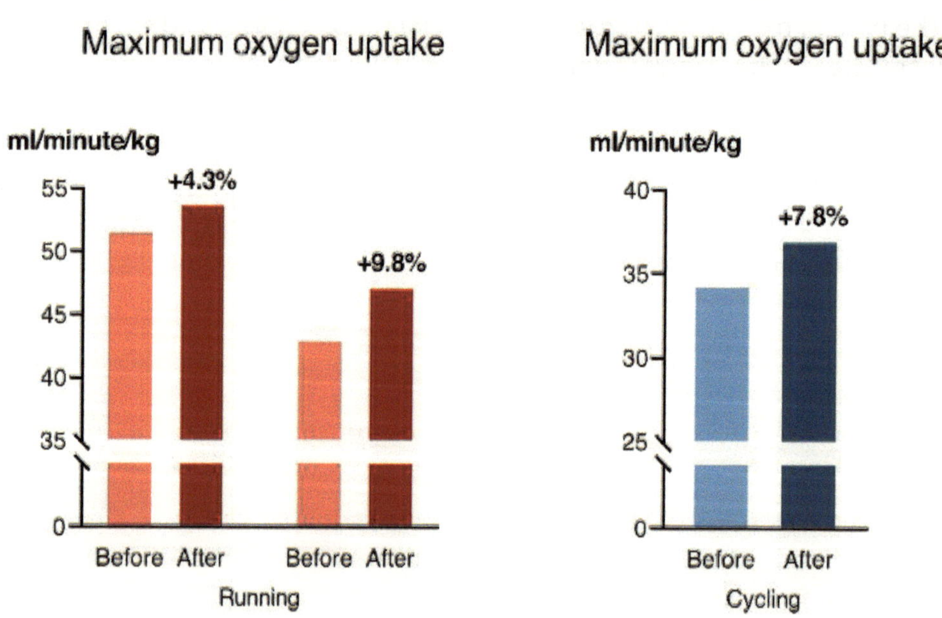

Figure 4. Effect 10-20-30 training on maximum oxygen uptake in two groups of both female and male runners (left) and in a group of men aged 55-65 years performing the training by cycling (right). It is clear that the 10-20-30 training led to marked improvements in maximum oxygen uptake.

Maximum oxygen uptake

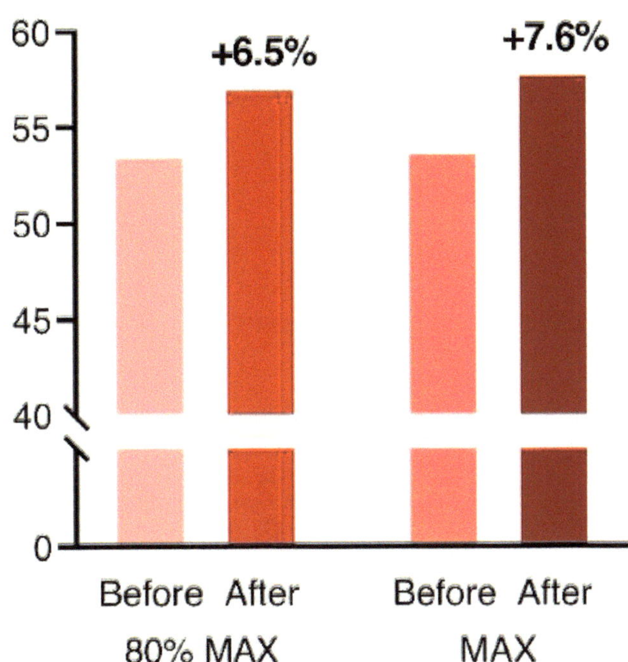

Figure 5. Effect 10-20-30 training on maximum oxygen uptake in two groups of trained runners where one group did maximally during the 10-second intervals (MAX), whereas the other group did only 80% of maximal effort (80%MAX). Note that both groups had major and the same improvement in maximum oxygen uptake.

10-20-30 training does increase performance

Trained runners who completed the 7 weeks of 10-20-30 training improved their time for a 1,500-meter run with 23 seconds and a 5-km run with 49 seconds (see Figure 6). It should be mentioned that a group (a so-called control group) that continued their normal training in the same period did not have any changes in performance. In another study, recreational runners completing 8 weeks of 10-20-30 training, with a reduction in training volume from about 15 to 11 km per week, improved their performance in a 1,000-meter run by 10 seconds (see Figure 6). Also doing 10-20-30 cycling does improve performance. A group of men aged 55-65 improved performance during a cycle test by 12% (see Figure 6).

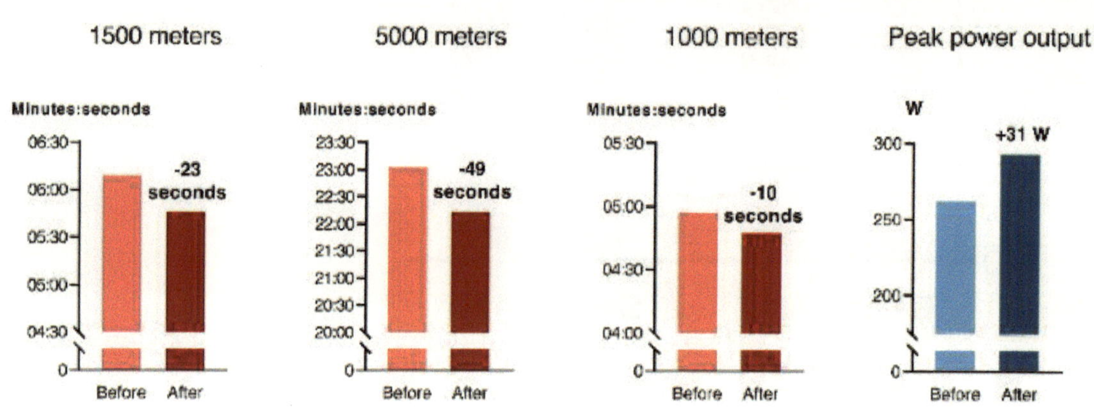

Figure 6. Effect of 10-20-30 training for trained runners on performance in a 1500-meter, a 5000 meter run, 1000 meter run (right) and in a group of men aged 55-65 years performing the 10-20-30 training by cycling (right). Note that all the participants had marked improvements.

Like for the maximum oxygen uptake, the group of runners performing 10-20-30 training only doing 80% of maximal effort during the 10-second intervals had the same improvement in performance during a 5-km run as the group doing maximal effort during the 10-second intervals (see Figure 7).

5000 meters

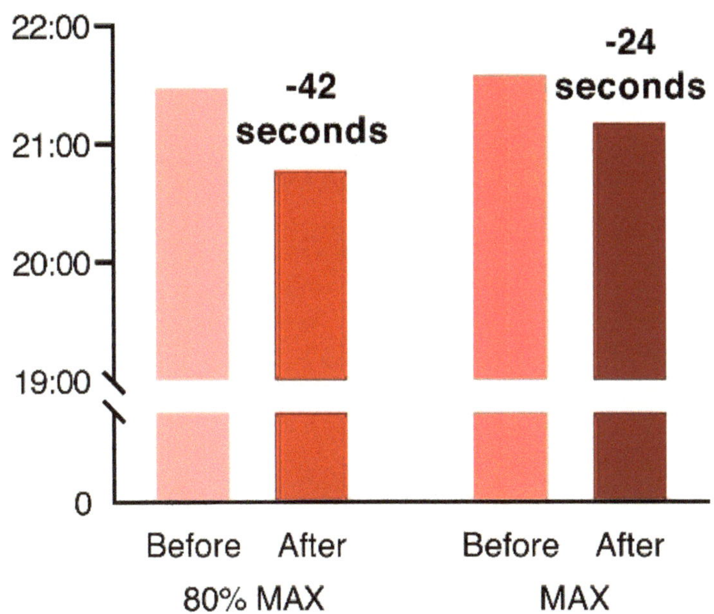

Figure 7. Effect 10-20-30 training on performance during a 5-km run in two groups of trained runners where one group did maximally during the 10-second intervals (MAX), whereas the other group did only 80% of maximal effort (80%MAX). Note that both groups had almost the same improvement in performance.

Measure your improvements

You do not need expensive equipment, if you want to follow yourself and measure your improvements. You can easily measure the effect of the 10-20-30 training.

If you are running, a simple way to evaluate the progress is to select a fixed test route or distance. It could be 1, 3 or 5 km depending on your preference. The distance does not need to be measured accurately. What is important is that it is the same route every time. The route should not have any sharpening turns that can disturb your rhythm. Neither should there be obstacles, such as traffic lights. You have to complete the distance as fast as possible each time, and if you do spent less time, you have improved.

On the bike, you select a standard load, e.g. 200 W, and you cycle at a frequency of 70 revolutions per minute as long as possible. When you are not able to maintain the

"The 10-20-30 training has been fun and inspiring, and sometimes hard, but I think it has been very rewarding"

Male, 44 years

frequency, i.e. the frequency drops below 65 revolutions per minute, you stop and the total exercise time represents the test result. The longer the better performance.

Typically, you can test yourself every 5th week.

Measuring resting heart rate

There are other simple ways you can determine whether you have improved. You can measure your heart rate at rest. The resting heart rate is how often the heart beats in a minute. The heart rate should be measured after you have been lying still for 5 minutes either by a heart rate monitor or manually by counting number of heart beats. The pulse can be obtained on the underside of the wrist or on the side of the neck. When you have found the pulse, you may count in 30 seconds and multiply the number by two to get the resting heart rate expressed in beats per minute. After a period of 10-20-30 training the resting heart rate becomes lower. This means that if your resting heart rate has dropped, then you are in better form.

Table 3 shows changes in resting heart rate for runners that for 7 weeks performed the 10-20-30 training twice in a week. Obviously, all the runners had lower resting heart rate after the 10-20-30 training period.

Table 3. Heart rate at rest for trained runners before and after a 7-week period with 10-20-30 training.

		Resting heart rate (beats/minute)	
Sex	Age (years)	Before	After
Women	24	77	73
Women	39	69	65
Women	56	70	68
Man	39	63	52
Man	69	66	61

10-20-30 training does lower blood pressure

There are two types of blood pressure. The systolic and diastolic blood pressure. The systolic blood pressure, also called stroke pressure, is the pressure that can be measured in the blood vessels, when the heart has contracted and pushed the blood into the blood vessels. The diastolic pressure, also called resting pressure, is the lowest pressure that can be measured in the blood vessels when the heart relaxes between two strokes. Ideally, systolic and diastolic blood pressure is around 120 and 80 mmHg, respectively. Ones talk about high blood pressure (hypertension), when the systolic blood pressure is above 140 mmHg and the diastolic blood pressure is above 90 mmHg. An elevated blood pressure may lead to serious cardiovascular diseases, such as blood clot in the brain and the heart as well heart and kidney failure.

After a 7-week 10-20-30 training period of trained runners, the systolic blood pressure was 5 mmHg lower (see Figure 8). Such a decrease reduces the risk of having cardiovascular problems by about 10-15 percent. There was no change in the diastolic blood pressure, but it was already optimal prior to the 10-20-30 training period. Thus, after the training period the participants´ blood pressure was 122 and 76 mmHg respectively, which are almost perfect.

The 10-20-30 training has an even greater effect of blood pressure of people with elevated blood pressure (hypertensive) as described on page 73.

Blood pressure gauges

Blood pressure gauges (see photo) are available in several different variants. Most are clinically validated and make accurate measurements.

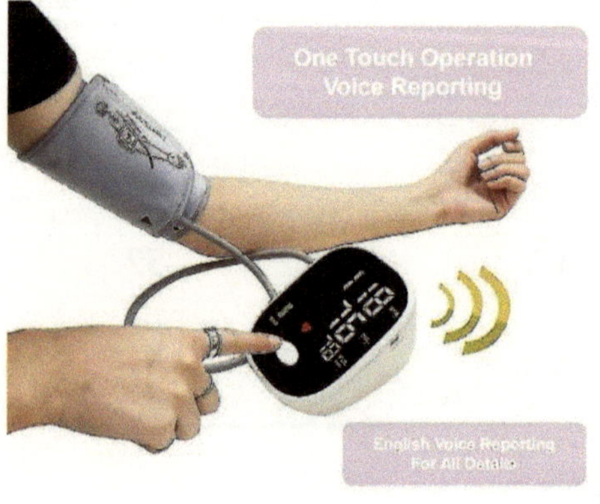

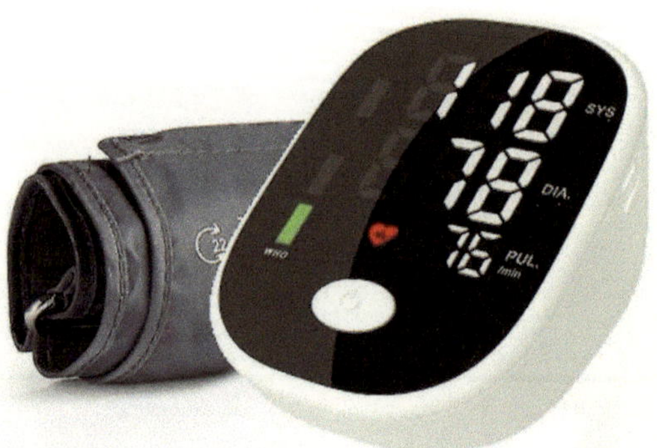

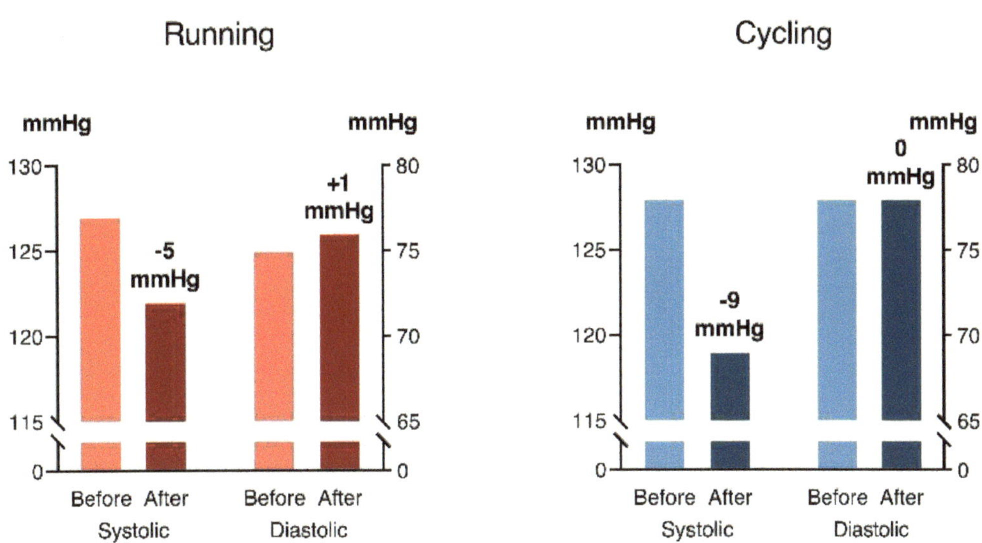

Figure 8. Effect of 10-20-30 training of trained runners (right) and in a group of men aged 55-65 years performing the training cycling (right) on systolic and diastolic blood pressure. Note that the systolic blood pressure in both groups decreased significant, which reduced the risk of cardiovascular diseases markedly.

Measurement of blood pressure

A simple way to get an idea of the effect of 10-20-30 training on your health is to measure blood pressure. However, it requires a blood pressure device, which you may buy at the Internet. The cheapest costs approximately 40 USD. When you measure blood pressure, it is important that you do it at the same time of the day. Sit down at a table, put the blood pressure cuff (see photo) around the upper arm and place the arm on the table. Relax for 5 minutes before you measure blood pressure. Take three measurements to make sure that you actually measure the resting blood pressure. If the measurements drop a lot from the first to the third, rest 5 minutes more, and then make three new measurements.

10-20-30 training does reduce blood cholesterol

After a 7-week 10-20-30 training period of trained runners the total amount of cholesterol in the blood was reduced by 10 percent (see Figure 9).

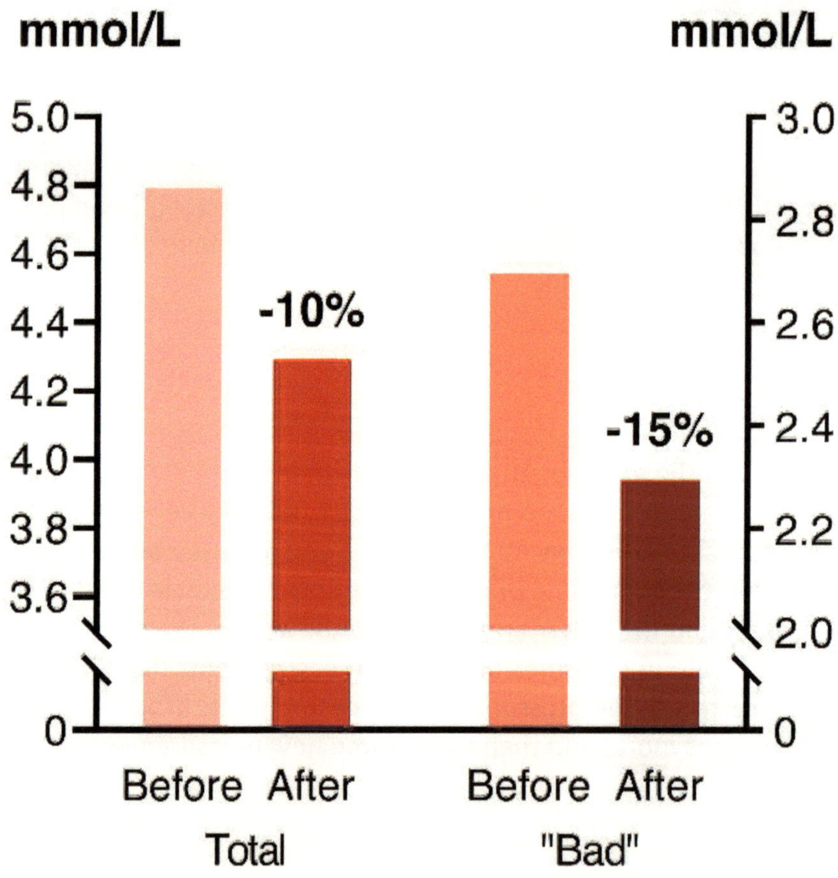

Figure 9. Effect of 7 weeks 10-20-30 training of trained runners on the amount of total (left) and 'bad' cholesterol (right) in the blood. The total cholesterol and bad cholesterol fell, which was extremely positive for the runners´ health.

Cholesterol is one of body fats and is important for building body cells and for the formation of certain hormones. The amount of cholesterol in the blood is depending on diet, training and production of cholesterol in the body. Cholesterol is bound to some special proteins, called lipoproteins, which carries cholesterol in the body. There are different types of lipoproteins. Low Density Lipoprotein (LDL) binds 60-70 percent of the body's total cholesterol. Cholesterol bound to LDL is often referred to as the 'bad' cholesterol, as it enhances the probability that fat is deposited on the inside of the blood vessels and gives atherosclerosis,

Cholesterol bound to High Density Lipoprotein (HDL) is often called the 'good' cholesterol because it transports cholesterol from the blood vessels to the liver, where cholesterol can be excreted. HDL typically binds 20-25 percent off the body's total cholesterol.

The amount of LDL-bound cholesterol in blood went from 2.7 to 2.3 millimoles (mmol) per litre in trained runners after 7 weeks of 10-20-30 training (see Figure 9). A fall in LDL-bound cholesterol of 1 mmol per liter can reduce the risk of getting a cardiovascular disease with approximately 25% regardless of the initial level, thus, the decrease of 0.4 mmol per liter reduced the risk of getting cardiovascular disease by more than 10 percent in these already trained people.

10-20-30 training does reduce body fat and increase muscle mass

10-20-30 training does reduce body fat. In a study with recreational runners conducting 10-20-30 training twice a week and one prolonged run a week, the participants lost 3.1 kg of fat in 8 weeks (see Figure 10), although the volume of training was reduced. They also increased the lean body mass with 2.7 kg (see Figure 11). Similarly, a group of middle-aged men lost 1.7 kg of fat with 6 weeks of 10-20-30 cycle training and has a small gain in lean body mass (see Figures 10 & 11).

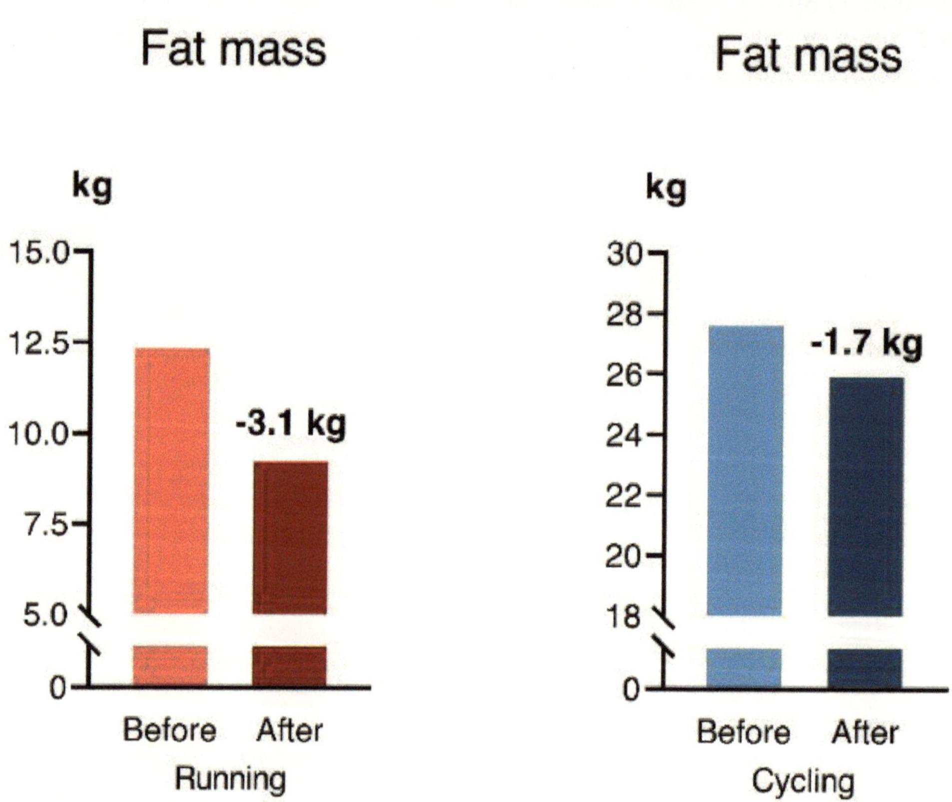

Figure 10. Effect of 10-20-30 training on fat mass for trained runners (left) and middle aged men cycling (right). Note that both groups had a significant loss of fat.

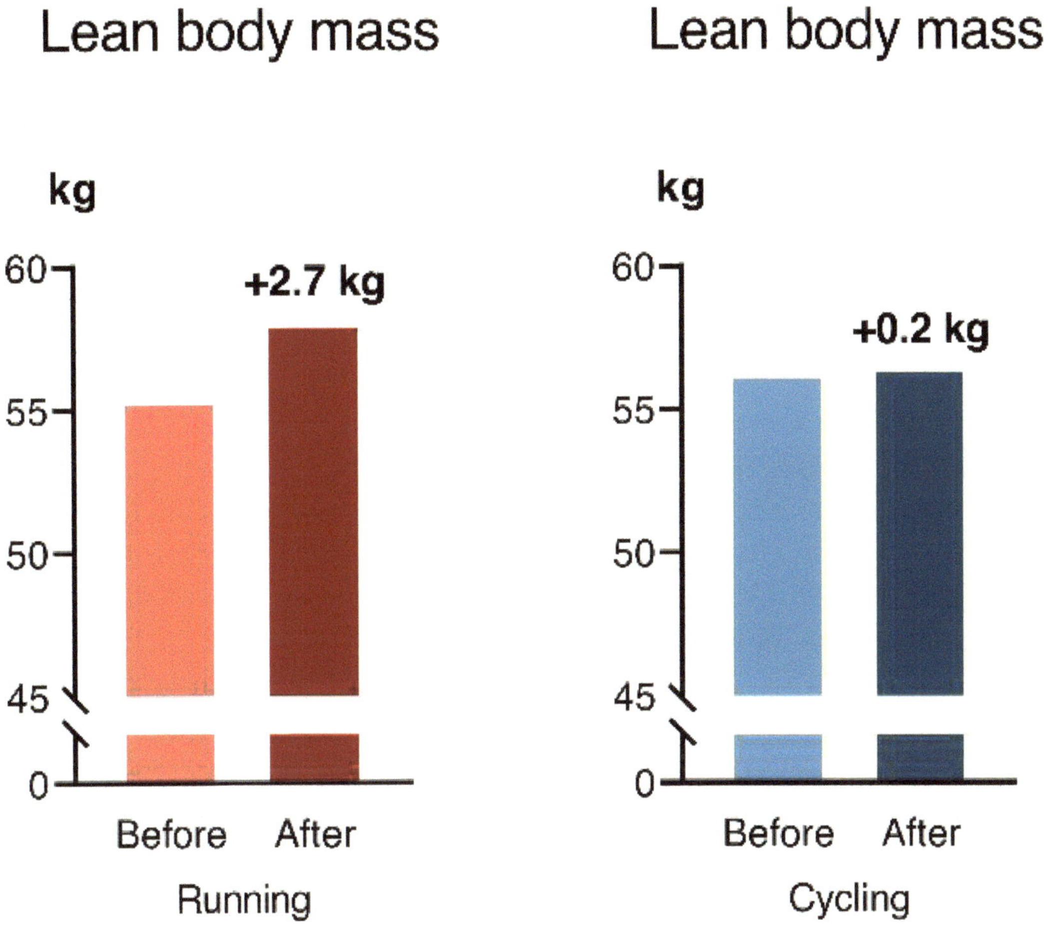

Lean body mass

Lean body mass

Figure 11. Effect of 10-20-30 training on lean body mass for trained runners (left) and middle aged men cycling (right). Note that both groups had a significant gain in muscle mass.

Synopsis – effect of 10-20-30 training

10-20-30 training not only improves performance and maximum oxygen uptake, it does also give a huge health boost even for well-trained people. One simply lowers fat mass, gets lower blood pressure and less harmful fat in the blood when doing 10-20-30 training. The explanation is that the intense part of training leads to a great activation of both the cardiovascular system and muscles. Thus, the heart is highly stimulated and at the same time, many muscle fibers are activated.

I've been exercising three times per week using 10 20 30 for the past 2 1/2 years. I have had very high blood pressure and high cholesterol for many years. A few years ago I was put on three different blood pressure drugs, which lowered my systolic to the mid 130's. Over the course of time using 10 20 30 it has further decreased to the low to mid 120's, sometimes dropping even further. My diastolic has always remained between 50 and 70. My cholesterol was over 250, sometimes down as low as 215. My first appointment with my family physician after beginning 10 20 30 revealed a major drop in cholesterol to 175 and has remained in that area ever since.

I just wanted to thank you for developing this routine as it has obviously been very beneficial to me.

Best to you

Male, USA

Beginner

When you have not been exercising before, or it is a long time ago, I will make sure you get the best possible start, i.e. that you do not get overloaded. If you are running, you need to make sure that you have proper running shoes. They do not need to be expensive and advanced. You have to select running shoes that suits you and which feels good. However, be aware, that running shoes are divided into three different types depending on your running style, i.e. how your foot is positioned when you are running: over pronation, neutral or supination. Running shoes have been developed to each of the three types of running style. If you are not sure which running style you have, then many sports stores offer a free running style test, which takes approximately 20 minutes. If you are cycling on you own bike in nature, you just need to have proper shoes that fits the bike. On a bike in a fitness center, most shoes will fit.

The next pages present programmes, which ensures you get the necessary progress in the right tempo. There is a programme for training once a week and one for training twice during a week. It is important that you follow the plan. It is beneficial if you make a deal with you selves or a friend to follow the program. Should it happen that that you miss a training session, it is important that you complete all sessions in the following week. Or even better that you conduct one extra session. However, do not train two days in a row.

The programmes presented are used both for running and cycling. When you are cycling, you should aim at a frequency between 60 and 80 revolutions per minute.

The programme shows the speed/intensity for 30- (blue), 20- (green) and 10- (red) seconds periods. As you get in better shape, the speed/intensity within the various categories will increase. The programme does also provide suggestions of when to test your selves.

The velocities/loadings are relative and given as:

	Running	Cycling
1	Walking	No load
2	Jogging	Low load
3	Running at a slow pace	Low/moderate load
4	Running at a moderate pace	Moderate load
5	Running at high speed	Moderate/high load
6	Sprinting	High load

Beginner – training once a week

Table 4 shows a programme for the beginner, who wants to train once a week. You may add the actual number of the weeks and make a cross when you have completed a session. If you want to avoid writing in the book, you may copy the form and hang it up.

Table 4. Program beginner training once a week.

	Training	Week*	Intensity # 30 20 10
Week 1	5 min warm-up 1x5min 10-20-30		1 2 4
Week 2	5 min warm-up 1x5min 10-20-30		1 2 4
Week 3	5 min warm-up 2x5min 10-20-30 Recovery 3 min		1 2 4
Week 4	5 min warm-up 2x5min 10-20-30 Recovery 3 min		1 2 5
Week 5	5 min warm-up 2x5min 10-20-30 Recovery 3 min		1 2 5
Week 6	5 min warm-up 2x5min 10-20-30 Recovery 4 min		1 3 5
Week 7	5 min warm-up 2x5min 10-20-30 Recovery 4 min		1 3 5
Week 8	5 min warm-up 2x5min 10-20-30 Recovery 4 min		1 4 5

Week 9	5 min warm-up 2x5min 10-20-30 Recovery 4 min		1 4 6
Week 10	Test (1 km run or 6 min cycle) and 1x5 min 10-20-30		1 4 6
Week 11	5 min warm-up 2x5min 10-20-30 Recovery 4 min		1 4 6
Week 12	5 min warm-up 2x5min 10-20-30 Recovery 4 min		1 4 6
Week 13	5 min warm-up 2x5min 10-20-30 Recovery 4 min		2 4 6
Week 14	5 min warm-up 2x5min 10-20-30 Recovery 4 min		2 4 6
Week 15	5 min warm-up 2x5min 10-20-30 Recovery 3 min		2 4 6
Week 16	Test (1 km run or 6 min cycle) and 1x5 min 10-20-30		2 4 6
Week 17	5 min warm-up 3x5min 10-20-30 Recovery 4 min		2 4 6
Week 18	5 min warm-up 3x5min 10-20-30		2 4 6

	Recovery 3 min		
Week 19	5 min warm-up 3x5min 10-20-30 Recovery 3 min		2 4 6
Week 20	5 min warm-up 3x5min 10-20-30 Recovery 3 min		2 4 6
Week 21	5 min warm-up 3x5min 10-20-30 Recovery 3 min		2 4 6
Week 22	Test (1 km run or 6 min cycle) and 2x5 min 10-20-30 Recovery 3 min		2 4 6
Week 23	5 min warm-up 3x5min 10-20-30 Recovery 2 min		2 4 6
Week 24	5 min warm-up 3x5min 10-20-30 Recovery 2 min		2 4 6
Week 25	5 min warm-up 4x5min 10-20-30 Recovery 3 min		2 4 6
Week 26	5 min warm-up 4x5min 10-20-30 Recovery 3 min		2 4 6
Week 27	5 min warm-up 4x5min 10-20-30		2 4 6

	Recovery 3 min			
Week 28	Test (1 km run or 6 min cycle) and 2x5 min 10-20-30 Recovery 3 min		2 4 6	
Week 29	5 min warm-up 4x5min 10-20-30 Recovery 2 min		2 4 6	
Week 30	5 min warm-up 4x5min 10-20-30 Recovery 2 min		2 4 6	
Week 31	5 min warm-up 4x5min 10-20-30 Recovery 2 min		2 4 6	
Week 32	5 min warm-up 4x5min 10-20-30 Recovery 2 min		2 4 6	
Week 33	5 min warm-up 4x5min 10-20-30 Recovery 2 min		2 4 6	
Week 34	5 min warm-up 4x5min 10-20-30 Recovery 2 min		2 4 6	
Week 35	Test (1-2 km) or Training (2 x 10-20-30 Recovery 3 min)		2 4 6	
Week 36	5 min warm-up 4x5min 10-20-30 Recovery 2 min		2 4 6	

* Enter the weeks according to when you start the training period.

Beginner - training twice a week

Table 5 (see page 50) shows a programme if you are beginner and want to do to two 10-20-30-training sessions a week. One of the session could be in the weekend, but the training can also be conducted two week days, they just have to be separated by a day for recovery. Below is a detail description to guide you through the programme (blue text is for cycling).

You build slowly up not to get overloaded. When you have done the program, you will be able to continue to the programs for trained presented on page 54. The programme can be conducted both running and cycling (blue). Follow the program below carefully (for a schematic overview see Table 5; page 50).

Week 1

Session 1: You must get started without being overloaded. For the first 10 minutes you switch between walking and jog or when cycling between no load and low load. It may change every minute, but if it is too strenuous, you may switch every 30 seconds. After 10 minutes, you start with the 10-20-30 training for 5 minutes. In the 30 seconds you walk/no load, in the 20 seconds you jog/low load and in the 10 seconds you run at moderate speed/moderate load.

Session 2: You continue with the modest loading. The training session is similar to session 1.

Week 2

Session 3: Now you should be ready to extend the 10-20-30 workout. You start again with the 10 minutes of switching between walking and jogging or when cycling between no load and moderate load. Next, 10-20-30 workouts for 2 x 5 minutes separated by a break of 4 minutes stretching legs and body. In the 30 seconds walking/no load, in the 20 seconds, you jog/low load, and in the 10 seconds, you run at moderate speed/loading.

Training 4: You continue with the extended 10-20-30 workout. The training is similar to session 3.

Week 3

Session 5: You need to do a little more in the warm up. In addition, you have to get used to run at a higher speed/higher loading and have a shorter break between intervals. You start with 10 minutes alternating between jogging/low loads for 2 minutes and walking/no load for 1 minute. Next, 10-20-30 workouts for 2 x 5 minutes separated by a 3-minute break. In the 30 seconds, you walk/no load, in the 20 seconds you jog/low load and in the 10 seconds, you run at high speed/high load.

Session 6: You continue at the higher speeds/loading. The session is similar to session 5.

Week 4

Session 7: You should now run a little faster than jog/increase the low load in the 20-seconds intervals and have a longer break between intervals. You start with 10 minutes, where you alternately between jogging/low load for 2 minutes and walking/no load for 1 minute. Then, 10-20-30 workout for 2 x 5 minutes separated by a 4-minute break. In the 30 seconds, you walk/no load, in the 20 seconds you now run at moderate speed/load, i.e. a little faster/higher load than you usually do and in the 10 seconds, you run at high speed/high load.

Session 8: You continue at the higher speeds/loads. The training is similar to session 7.

Week 5

Session 9: You continue with the higher speeds/loads, and you need to do a bit more during the warming-up. You start with 10 minutes, where you alternately jog/low load for 3 minutes and walk/no load for 1 minute. Then 10-20-30 training for 2 x 5 minutes separated by a 4-minute break. In the 30 seconds, you walk/no load, in the 20 seconds, you run at moderate speed/moderate load and in the 10 seconds, you run at high speed/high load.

Session 10: You continue at the higher speeds/loads. The training is similar to session 9.

Week 6

Session 11: You have now been training for 5 weeks. Want to test yourself? If you are running, you may find a suitable route of around 1 km and record the time to complete it, or if you are cycling, you choose a moderate loading and see how long you can maintain a frequency of a 70 revolutions per minute. Start with warming up for 10 minutes, alternate between jogging/low load for 3 minutes and 1 minute of walking/no load. After the test, you can choose to rest or do 1 x 10-20-30 at the speeds you used in session 9. If you do not want to be tested, you can do the training described in session 9.

Training 12: How did the test go? If you were able to run all the time, or keep the pace on the cycle, it is very good. Now you also have to run or cycle with low loading for the 30-second intervals, and do some more in the warming up, where you do 2 minutes jogging/low load followed by 3 minutes of moderate speed/moderate load. Then, 10-20-30 workouts for 2 x 5 minutes are separated by a 4-minute break. In the 30 seconds, you now jog/low load, and in the 20-seconds intervals, you run at a moderate speed/cycle with moderate load and for the 10 seconds you run at high speed/cycle at high load.

Session 13: You continue with the higher speeds/loads. The training is similar to session 12.

Week 7

Session 14: You continue increasing the speeds/loads. In the warm-up you do 2 minutes jogging/low load followed by 3 minutes of moderate speed/moderate load. Then, 10-20-30 workouts for 2 x 5 minutes separated by a 4-minute break. In the 30-second intervals, you jog/low load, in the 20-second intervals you run/cycle at a moderate speed/moderate load and for the 10 seconds you run at high speed/high load.

Session 15: You may be able to speed up/increase the load during the 20-second intervals and reduce the recovery time between the 10-20-30 intervals. You start with the 5-minute warm up as in session 14. Next, 10-20-30 workouts for 2 x 5 minutes separated by a break of 3 minutes. In the 30 seconds, you jog/low load, in the 20 seconds you run/cycle at moderate speed/load, but now slightly higher than in session 14, and in the 10- second intervals you run/cycle at high speed/high load.

Week 8

Session 16: You continue at the higher speeds/loads. The training is similar to session 15.

Session 17: You extend the 10-20-30 workout, but have longer breaks between intervals. You start with warm-up doing 2 minutes jogging/low load followed by 3 minutes of moderate speed/moderate load. Next, 10-20-30- training for 3 x 5 minutes separated by 4- minute breaks. In the 30 seconds you jog/low load, in the 20 seconds you run/cycle at moderate speed/moderate load (as in training 16), and in the 10-second intervals you run at high speed/high load.

Week 9

Training 18: You continue with the extended training. The training is similar to session 17.

Session 19: You continue with the higher speeds/loads and now a shorter break between the intervals. You do 2 minutes jogging/low load followed by 3 minutes of moderate speed/moderate load as warm up. Then, 10-20-30 workouts for 3 x 5 minutes separated by breaks of 3 minutes. In the 30 seconds, you jog/low load, in the 20 seconds you run/cycle at moderate speed/moderate load and for 10 seconds you run/cycle at high speed/high load.

Week 10

Session 20: You continue at the higher speeds/loads. The training is similar as session 19.

Session 21: You have now trained well for 10 weeks. Want to test yourself (again)? You do the same route (around 1 km) as in week 6 and record the time it takes to complete or on the bike, the same load as in week 6, and see how long you can maintain the frequency of 70 revolutions per minute. Start with warming up for 10 minutes, alternate between jogging/low load for 3 minutes and 1 minute of walking/no load. After the test, you can choose to stop or do 2 x 10-20-30 with the speeds/loads you used in training 19 separated by 3-minute break. If you do not want to be tested, you can do the training as in session 19.

Week 11

Training 22: How did the test go? Have you improved by more than 10 seconds from the test in week 6, it is good. Now you will reduce the break between intervals. You start with 2 minutes jogging/low load followed by 3 minutes of moderate speed/moderate load as warm up. Next, 10-20-30 workouts for 3 x 5 minutes separated by 2-minute breaks. In the 30 seconds, you jog/low load, in the 20 seconds you run/cycle at moderate speed/moderate load, and in the 10-second intervals, you run at high speed/high load.

Session 23: You must now run even faster in the 10 seconds. You start with 2 minutes jogging/low load followed by 3 minutes of moderate speed/moderate load as warm up. Then, 10-20-30 workouts for 3 x 5 minutes separated by 2-minute breaks. In the 30 seconds, you jog/low load, in the 20-second intervals you run/cycle at a moderate speed/moderate load, and for 10 seconds you do sprint, i.e. runs at the highest possible speed, or do maximal on the cycle by increasing both the load and the frequency.

Week 12

Session 24: You continue at the higher speeds/loads. The training is similar to session 23.

Session 25: You continue with the higher speeds/loads and shorter breaks in between 10-20-30 intervals. The training is similar to training 23.

Week 13

Session 26: You continue with the higher speeds/loads and shorter breaks. The training is the same as session 23.

Session 27: Now expand the 10-20-30 training and have a longer break between the intervals. You do 2 minutes jogging/low load followed by 3 minutes of moderate speed/moderate load as warm up. Next, 10-20-30 workouts for 4 x 5 minutes separated by breaks of 3 minutes. In the 30 seconds, you jog/low load, in the 20 seconds you run/cycle at moderate speed/moderate load, and in the 10 seconds, you sprint (on the bike high load and high frequency).

Week 14

Session 28: You continue with the extended 10-20-30 program. The training is similar to training 27.

Session 29: You continue with the extended 10-20-30 program and increase the speed/load of the 20 seconds. The training is similar to training 27, though at a slightly higher speed/load in the 20 seconds, i.e. you start with 2 minutes jogging/low load followed by 3 minutes of moderate speed/moderate load as warm up. Next, 10-20-30 training in 4 x 5 minutes separated by 3-minute breaks. In the 30 seconds jog/low load, in the 20 seconds you run/cycle at moderate/load but higher speed/load, and in the 10 seconds you sprint.

Week 15

Session 30: You continue at the higher speeds/loads. The training is similar to session 29.

Session 31: You have now trained well for 15 weeks. Want to test yourself again? When running use the same route, or on the bike the same load, as in week 6 and 12 and record the time. Start with warming up for 10 minutes, alternate between jogging/low load for 3 minutes and 1 minute of walking/no load. After the test you can choose to stop or make 2 x 10-20-30 with the speeds/loads you used in session 29 separated by a break of 3 minutes. If you do not want to be tested, you can do the training described in session 29.

Week 16

Session 32: How did the test go? If you were able to run at least 1 km in a good pace without pausing, or cycling for more than 10 minutes, you shave done very well. You may continue with the programme for trained "Training twice a week" on page 54. You may also continue with this programme. Then, you should complete the training as in session 29.

Session 33: Train as in session 29.

Weeks 17-20

Sessions 34-40: Now you have reached the final step of the 10-20-30 training programme for beginners. Hope you have enjoyed it. As usual you warm-up with 2 minutes jogging/low load followed by 3 minutes of moderate speed/moderate load. The training continues with higher speed/loads in the 20-second intervals and with a shorter break between the 5-minute intervals. You do, 4 x 5 minutes separated by 2-minute breaks. In the 30 seconds, you jog or cycle with low load, in the 20 seconds you run/cycle at a moderate speed with slightly higher speed/load, and in the 10-second intervals, you sprint.

Week 21

Session 41: You have now been training well for 20 weeks. Want to test yourself (again)? You should to the route you have been doing previous or cycle at the intensity you have used in the previous tests , and record the time to complete the test .You do the warm-up as before the previous tests, i.e. warming up for 10 minutes, alternate between jogging/low load for 3 minutes and 1 minute of walking/no load.

After the test, you can choose to stop or make 2 x 10-20-30 at the speeds/loads you used in session 40 separated by a 2-minute break. If you do not want to be tested, you can train as in session 40.

Training 42: How did the test go? Have you improved by more than 15 seconds, it is really good. Now you are no longer beginner and should switch to the programmes for trained. If you want to train twice a week go to programme in Table 6 (page 54) and start with week 6, if you want to train three times a week then go to Table 7 (page 57) and start with week 6.

Table 5. Program beginner training twice a week.

	First session	Second session	Week*	Intensity
	Tuesday/Wednesday/Thursday	Friday/Saturday/Sunday		#
				30 20 10
Week 1	5 min warm-up	5 min warm-up		1 2 4
	1x5min 10-20-30	1x5min 10-20-30		1 2 4
Week 2	5 min warm-up	5 min warm-up		1 2 4
	2x5min 10-20-30	2x5min 10-20-30		1 2 4
	Recovery 4 min	Recovery 4 min		
Week 3	5 min warm-up	5 min warm-up		1 2 5
	2x5min 10-20-30	2x5min 10-20-30		1 2 5
	Recovery 3 min	Recovery 3 min		
Week 4	5 min warm-up	5 min warm-up		1 3 5
	2x5min 10-20-30	2x5min 10-20-30		1 3 5
	Recovery 4 min	Recovery 4 min		
Week 5	5 min warm-up	5 min warm-up		1 4 5
	2x5min 10-20-30	2x5min 10-20-30		1 4 5
	Recovery 4 min	Recovery 4 min		
Week 6	Test (1 km run or 6 min cycle)	5 min warm-up		1 4 5
	and	2x5min 10-20-30		2 4 5
	1x5 min 10-20-30	Recovery 4 min		

Week 7	5 min warm-up 2x5min 10-20-30 Recovery 4 min	5 min warm-up 2x5min 10-20-30 Recovery 4 min		2	4	5 2 4 5
Week 8	5 min warm-up 2x5min 10-20-30 Recovery 3 min	5 min warm-up 2x5min 10-20-30 Recovery 3 min		2	4	5 2 4 5
Week 9	5 min warm-up 3x5min 10-20-30 Recovery 4 min	5 min warm-up 3x5min 10-20-30 Recovery 4 min		2	4	5 2 4 5
Week 10	5 min warm-up 3x5min 10-20-30 Recovery 3 min	5 min warm-up 3x5min 10-20-30 Recovery 3 min		2	4	5 2 4 5
Week 11	Test (1-3 km run or 6 min cycle) and 2x5 min 10-20-30	5 min warm-up 3x5min 10-20-30 Recovery 2 min		2	4	5 2 4 5
Week 12	5 min warm-up 3x5min 10-20-30 Recovery 2 min	5 min warm-up 3x5min 10-20-30 Recovery 2 min		2	4	6 2 4 6
Week 13	5 min warm-up 3x5min 10-20-30 Recovery 2 min	5 min warm-up 3x5min 10-20-30 Recovery 2 min		2	4	6 2 4 6
Week 14	5 min warm-up 4x5min 10-20-30 Recovery 3 min	5 min warm-up 4x5min 10-20-30 Recovery 3 min		2	4	6 2 4 6
Week 15	5 min warm-up 4x5min 10-20-30 Recovery 3 min	5 min warm-up 4x5min 10-20-30 Recovery 3 min		2	4	6 2 4 6

Week 16	Test (1-3 km run or 6 min cycle) and 2x5 min 10-20-30 Recovery 3 min	5 min warm-up 4x5min 10-20-30 Recovery 3 min		2 4 6 2 4 6
Week 17	5 min warm-up 4x5min 10-20-30 Recovery 2 min	5 min warm-up 4x5min 10-20-30 Recovery 2 min		2 4 6 2 4 6
Week 18	5 min warm-up 4x5min 10-20-30 Recovery 2 min	5 min warm-up 4x5min 10-20-30 Recovery 2 min		2 4 6 2 4 6
Week 19	5 min warm-up 4x5min 10-20-30 Recovery 2 min	5 min warm-up 4x5min 10-20-30 Recovery 2 min		2 4 6 2 4 6
Week 20	5 min warm-up 4x5min 10-20-30 Recovery 2 min	5 min warm-up 4x5min 10-20-30 Recovery 2 min		2 4 6 2 4 6
Week 21	Test (1-3 km run or 6 min cycle) and 2x5 min 10-20-30 Recovery 2 min	5 min warm-up 4x5min 10-20-30 Recovery 2 min		2 4 6 2 4 6
Week 22	See program for "trained twice a week" (page 54)			

* Enter the weeks according to when you start the training period.

Trained

Even if you are used to run or cycle you should spend some time getting accustomed to the 10-20-30 training, so you do not get overloaded. It is mainly the 10 seconds of high intensity that can be stressful. Therefore, the first times you do the 10-second intervals you should only run or cycle slightly faster than normally. As you get used to the intensity during the 10 seconds, you increase the intensity, and it may eventually become a sprint.

During the first two weeks of the new training period, you may just substitute one of your training sessions with the 10-20-30 training. Then, you may choose to still have one training with prolonged moderate intensity exercise and do the 10-20-30 training at the other sessions.

How often will you train?

The rest of this chapter is divided into, whether you train twice or three times in a week. For three sessions per week there are two programs either 3 times 10-20-30 training per week (see page 57) or 2 x 10-20-30 training and one prolonged moderate intensity exercise training session a week (see page 60). In the last case, you may do 10-20-30 training on weekdays, when the time is limited, and then the longer session in the weekend, where you have more time.

The programs are developed with a lead-in period, where you become accustomed to the 10-20-30 training. Remember that you the first times should not do maximally in the 10-second periods, but simply increase the intensity after the 20-second with moderate pace. You may like to do a test before you start the 10-20-30 training program in order to be able to measure your progress. You can choose a distance, e.g. 3 km, if you are running, or a proper load, e.g. 200 W, on the bike, and then measure the time to complete the run or time to exhaustion on the bike.

The programs presented are used for both running and cycling. When you are cycling, you should aim at a frequency between 60 and 80 revolutions per minute.

Trained - 10-20-30 training twice a week

Table 6 (see page 54) shows a program if you are trained and want to do to two 10-20-30 training sessions in a week. The program have a lead-in phase where you get used to the 10-20-30 training. Remember that you are not supposed to do maximal the first times during the 10 seconds with high intensity, it is enough simply to increase the speed, if you are running, or the load on the bike after the 20-second moderate intensity. Before starting the training program, you can choose to conduct a test to measure your progress. If you are running you may choose a 3-km distance, and if you are biking you may chose a loading, which will exhaust you within about 10 minutes (you continue as long as the number of revolutions is not dropping significantly). It is just important, that you do the upcoming tests on the same route if running, and same loading if cycling.

One of the session could be in the weekend, but the training can also be conducted two week days, they just have to be separated by a day of recovery.

Table 6. Program for trained training twice a week.

	Session 1 Tuesday/Wednesday/Thursday	Session 2 Saturday/Sunday	Week*
Week 1	Test – run: 3 km – cycle: about 10 minutes	20 min moderate intensity 1x5min 10-20-30	
Week 2	20 min moderate intensity 1x5min 10-20-30	20 min moderate intensity 1x5min 10-20-30	
Week 3	15 min moderate intensity 2x5min 10-20-30 3 min recovery	15 min moderate intensity 2x5min 10-20-30	
Week 4	5 min moderate intensity 3x5min 10-20-30 3 min recovery	5 min moderate intensity 3x5min 10-20-30 3 min recovery	
Week 5	5 min moderate intensity 3x5min 10-20-30 3 min recovery	5 min moderate intensity 3x5min 10-20-30 3 min recovery	
Week 6	Test – run: 3 km – cycle: about 10 minutes	5 min moderate intensity 3x5min 10-20-30 3 min recovery	
Week 7	5 min moderate intensity 3x5min 10-20-30 3 min recovery	5 min moderate intensity 3x5min 10-20-30 2 min recovery	
Week 8	5 min moderate intensity 3x5min 10-20-30 2 min recovery	5 min moderate intensity 4x5min 10-20-30 3 min recovery	

Week 9	5 min moderate intensity 4x5min 10-20-30 3 min recovery	5 min moderate intensity 4x5min 10-20-30 3 min recovery	
Week 10	5 min moderate intensity 4x5min 10-20-30 3 min recovery	5 min moderate intensity 4x5min 10-20-30 3 min recovery	
Week 11	5 min moderate intensity 4x5min 10-20-30 2 min recovery	5 min moderate intensity 4x5min 10-20-30 2 min recovery	
Week 12	Test – run: 3 km – cycle: about 10 minutes	5 min moderate intensity 4x5min 10-20-30 2 min recovery	
Week 13	5 min moderate intensity 4x5min 10-20-30 2 min recovery	5 min moderate intensity 4x5min 10-20-30 2 min recovery	
Week 14	5 min moderate intensity 4x5min 10-20-30 2 min recovery	5 min moderate intensity 4x5min 10-20-30 2 min recovery	
Week 15	5 min moderate intensity 4x5min 10-20-30 2 min recovery	5 min moderate intensity 4x5min 10-20-30 2 min recovery	
Week 16	5 min moderate intensity 4x5min 10-20-30 2 min recovery	5 min moderate intensity 4x5min 10-20-30 2 min recovery	
Week 17	5 min moderate intensity 4x5min 10-20-30 2 min recovery	5 min moderate intensity 4x5min 10-20-30 2 min recovery	

| Week 18 | Test – run: 3 km

-cycle: about 10 minutes | 5 min moderate intensity

4x5min 10-20-30

2 min recovery | |

* Enter the weeks according to when you start the training period.

Trained – training three times a week

In this section, there are two programs depending on whether you would like to complete two 10-20-30 training sessions and a prolonged training session at moderate intensity once a week or you will do 10-20-30 training three times a week. Both are effective so you can freely choose. Both programs have a lead-in phase where you get used to the 10-20-30 training. Remember that you are not supposed to do maximal the first times during 10 seconds with high intensity, it is enough simply to increase the speed, if you are running, or the load on the bike after the 20-second moderate intensity. Before starting the training program, you can choose to complete a test to be able to measure your progress. If you are running you may choose a 5-km distance and if you are biking you may chose a loading, which will exhaust you within about 15 minutes (you continue until the number of revolutions is dropping significantly). It is just important that you do the upcoming tests on the same route if running, and same loading if cycling.

Table 7 and Table 8 (see page 60) shows programs for the trained doing three sessions a week without and with one prolonged moderate intensity session, respectively.

Table 7. Program for trained with 10-20-30 training three times a week.

	First session Monday/Tuesday	**Second session** Wednesday/Thursday	**Third session** Friday/Saturday/Sunday	**Week***
Week 1	Test – run: 5km -cycle: about 15 min	20 min moderate intensity 1x5min 10-20-30	Prolonged moderate intensity	
Week 2	20 min moderate intensity 1x5min 10-20-30	20 min moderate intensity 1x5min 10-20-30	Prolonged moderate intensity	
Week 3	15 min moderate intensity 2x5min 10-20-30 3 min recovery	15 min moderate intensity 2x5min 10-20-30 3 min recovery	Prolonged moderate intensity	
Week 4	10 min moderate intensity 3x5min 10-20-30	10 min moderate intensity 3x5min 10-20-30	10 min moderate intensity 3x5min 10-20-30	

	3 min recovery	3 min recovery	3 min recovery
Week 5	5-min warm-up 3x5min 10-20-30 2 min recovery	5-min warm-up 3x5min 10-20-30 2 min recovery	5-min warm-up 3x5min 10-20-30 2 min recovery
Week 6	Test – run: 5km -cycle: about 15 min or 3x5min 10-20-30 2 min recovery	5-min warm-up 3x5min 10-20-30 2 min recovery	5-min warm-up 3x5min 10-20-30 2 min recovery
Week 7	5-min warm-up 3x5min 10-20-30 2 min recovery	5-min warm-up 3x5min 10-20-30 2 min recovery	5-min warm-up 3x5min 10-20-30 2 min recovery
Week 8	5-min warm-up 3x5min 10-20-30 2 min recovery	5-min warm-up 4x5min 10-20-30 3 min recovery	5-min warm-up 4x5min 10-20-30 3 min recovery
Week 9	5-min warm-up 4x5min 10-20-30 3 min recovery	5-min warm-up 4x5min 10-20-30 3 min recovery	5-min warm-up 4x5min 10-20-30 3 min recovery
Week 10	5-min warm-up 4x5min 10-20-30 2 min recovery	5-min warm-up 4x5min 10-20-30 2 min recovery	5-min warm-up 4x5min 10-20-30 2 min recovery
Week 11	Test – run: 5km -cycle: about 15 min or 4x5min 10-20-30 2 min recovery	5-min warm-up 4x5min 10-20-30 2 min recovery	5-min warm-up 4x5min 10-20-30 2 min recovery

Week 12	5-min warm-up	5-min warm-up	5-min warm-up	
	4x5min 10-20-30	4x5min 10-20-30	4x5min 10-20-30	
	2 min recovery	2 min recovery	2 min recovery	
Week 13	5-min warm-up	5-min warm-up	5-min warm-up	
	4x5min 10-20-30	4x5min 10-20-30	4x5min 10-20-30	
	2 min recovery	2 min recovery	2 min recovery	
Week 14	5-min warm-up	5-min warm-up	5-min warm-up	
	4x5min 10-20-30	4x5min 10-20-30	4x5min 10-20-30	
	2 min recovery	2 min recovery	2 min recovery	
Week 15	5-min warm-up	5-min warm-up	5-min warm-up	
	4x5min 10-20-30	4x5min 10-20-30	4x5min 10-20-30	
	2 min recovery	2 min recovery	2 min recovery	
Week 16	Test – run: 5km	5-min warm-up	5-min warm-up	
	-cycle: about 15	4x5min 10-20-30	4x5min 10-20-30	
	min or	2 min recovery	2 min recovery	
	4x5min 10-20-30			
	2 min recovery			

*Enter the weeks according to when you start the training period.

Table 8. Program for trained with 10-20-30 training twice a week and a prolonged moderate intensity session a week.

	First session Monday/Tuesday	Second session Wednesday/Thursday	Third session Friday/Saturday/Sunday	Week*
Week 1	Test – run: 5km cycle: about 15 min	20 min moderate intensity 1x5min 10-20-30	Prolonged moderate intensity	
Week 2	20 min moderate intensity 1x5min 10-20-30	Prolonged moderate intensity	Prolonged moderate intensity	
Week 3	15 min moderate intensity 2x5min 10-20-30 3 min recovery	15 min moderate intensity 2x5min 10-20-30 3 min recovery	Prolonged moderate intensity	
Week 4	5-min warm-up 3x5min 10-20-30 3 min recovery	5-min warm-up 3x5min 10-20-30 3 min recovery	Prolonged moderate intensity	
Week 5	5-min warm-up 3x5min 10-20-30 3 min recovery	5-min warm-up 3x5min 10-20-30 3 min recovery	Prolonged moderate intensity	
Week 6	Test – run: 5km cycle: about 15 min or 3x5min 10-20-30 3 min recovery	5-min warm-up 3x5min 10-20-30 3 min recovery	Prolonged moderate intensity	
Week 7	5-min warm-up 3x5min 10-20-30 3 min recovery	5-min warm-up 3x5min 10-20-30 2 min recovery	Prolonged moderate intensity	

Week 8	5-min warm-up 3x5min 10-20-30 2 min recovery	5-min warm-up 3x5min 10-20-30 2 min recovery	Prolonged moderate intensity
Week 9	5-min warm-up 4x5min 10-20-30 3 min recovery	5-min warm-up 4x5min 10-20-30 3 min recovery	Prolonged moderate intensity
Week 10	5-min warm-up 4x5min 10-20-30 2 min recovery	5-min warm-up 4x5min 10-20-30 2 min recovery	Prolonged moderate intensity
Week 11	Test – run: 5km cycle: about 15 min or 4x5min 10-20-30 2 min recovery	5-min warm-up 4x5min 10-20-30 2 min recovery	Prolonged moderate intensity
Week 12	5-min warm-up 4x5min 10-20-30 2 min recovery	5-min warm-up 4x5min 10-20-30 2 min recovery	Prolonged moderate intensity
Week 13	5-min warm-up 4x5min 10-20-30 2 min recovery	5-min warm-up 4x5min 10-20-30 2 min recovery	Prolonged moderate intensity
Week 14	5-min warm-up 4x5min 10-20-30 2 min recovery	5-min warm-up 4x5min 10-20-30 2 min recovery	Prolonged moderate intensity
Week 15	5-min warm-up 4x5min 10-20-30 2 min recovery	5-min warm-up 4x5min 10-20-30 2 min recovery	Prolonged moderate intensity
Week 16	5-min warm-up 4x5min 10-20-30 2 min recovery	5-min warm-up 4x5min 10-20-30 2 min recovery	Prolonged moderate intensity

Week 17	5-min warm-up 4x5min 10-20-30 2 min recovery	Test – run: 5km cycle: about 15 min or 3x5min 10-20-30 3 min recovery	Prolonged moderate intensity	
Week 18	5-min warm-up 4x5min 10-20-30 2 min recovery	5-min warm-up 4x5min 10-20-30 2 min recovery	Prolonged moderate intensity	

* Enter the weeks according to when you start the training period.

Type 2 diabetes patients

Diabetes is one of the most common chronic diseases worldwide with more than 400 mill diagnosed, and as many with pre-diabetes with a significant risk of developing diabetes. Type 2 diabetes accounts for ~90% of the diabetes cases, and is characterized by a decreased insulin sensitivity leading to impaired glucose tolerance. It typically arises from a sedentary lifestyle, poor diet or genetic susceptibility.

Exercise training is effective in improving glycemic control in persons with type 2 diabetes, and is a cornerstone in the first line of treatment. The official exercise recommendations for people diagnosed with type 2 diabetes are a minimum of 150 minutes of physical activity per week. A life-style intervention with moderate-intensity training alone or including diet control can elicit a number of positive adaptations in patients with type 2 diabetes. Thus, scientific studies have observed valuable changes in glycemic control during training protocols consisting of moderate intensity training more than five days per week with 175-320 min exercise per week. However, such an extensive exercise setup may not be feasible due to "a lack of time" as reported as one of the most cited barriers for not engaging in physical exercise among patients with type 2 diabetes. In general, adherence to exercise training is lower within this group compared to the healthy population. Therefore, 10-20-30 training is optimal for these patients.

10-20-30 training of diabetes patients

The effect of a 10-week 10-20-30 cycle training intervention on diabetes patients was studied and compared to the effect of moderate intensity training recommended for diabetic patients. The patients were diagnosed with type 2 diabetes from 0.5 to 10 years

The 10-20-30 training group warmed up for 10 minutes with low intensity cycling and exercised according to the 10-20-30 training concept consisting of 3 x 5 minutes of cycling interspersed by 2 minutes of rest. In each 5-minute period the patients conducted five consecutive 1-minute intervals divided into 30, 20 and 10 seconds at low, moderate and maximal-intensity, respectively. The intensities were based on each subjects' individual perception. The 10-20-30 training was conducted three times a week.

The moderate-intensity training group trained according to the official exercise recommendations for patients with type 2 diabetes. The training consisted of 50 minutes moderate-intensity continuous cycling three times a week.

Figure 12 shows the heart rate response during the two types of training. It is clear that heart rate was significantly higher during the 10-20-30 training.

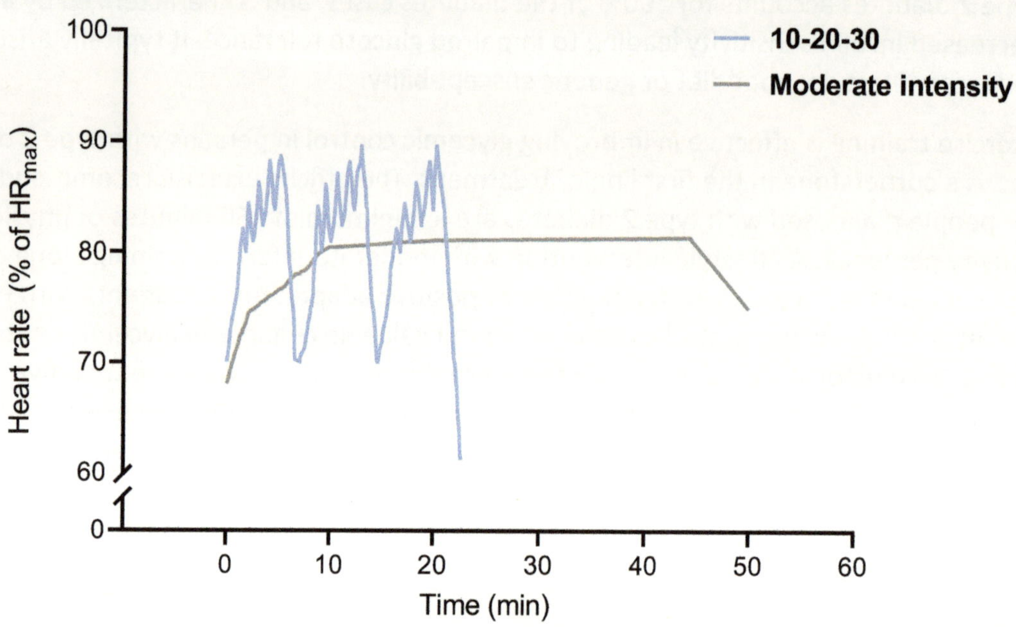

Figure 12. Heart rate for patients with type 2 diabetes during 10-20-30 training (blue) and moderate-intensity training (black). Note that the heart rate is much higher with 10-20-30 training.

The training was conducted in a fitness center. Compliance to training was 84% and 86% in the 10-20-30 and moderate intensity training group, respectively. Thus, the 10-20-30 and moderate-intensity training group completed on average 2.5 and 2.6 training sessions per week corresponding to a total of 25 and 26 training sessions, respectively.

Effect of 10-20-30 training on long-term blood glucose of diabetes patients

Long-term blood glucose, called HbA1c, is a term commonly used in relation to diabetes, it refers to glycated hemoglobin. It develops when hemoglobin (a protein within red blood cells that carries oxygen throughout your body) joins with glucose in the blood and becomes 'glycated'. It provides an overall picture of what our average blood sugar levels have been over a period of weeks/months. For people with diabetes this is important, as the higher the HbA1c the greater the risk of developing diabetes-related complications. The level of HbA1c also provide information about the condition of a person as shown in Table 9.

Table 9. The table shows how the concentration of HbA1c can indicate people with prediabetes or diabetes.

	HbA1c	
	mmol/mol	%
Normal	<42	<6
Pre-diabetes	42-47	6.0-6.4
Diabetes	>47	>6.4

All the diabetic patients in the study had HbA_{1c} values higher than 7% before the training intervention. After 10 weeks the 10-20-30 training group had a ~0.5% point reduction in HbA_{1c}, whereas no change was observed in the group doing moderate intensity training (see Figure 13), despite this group had an about 50% higher training volume. Thus, it appears that the 10-20-30 training is superior in the treatment of type 2 diabetes patients compared to moderate intensity training.

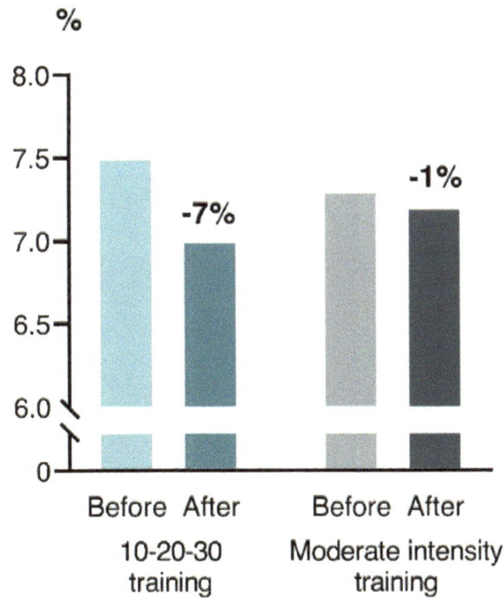

Figure 13. Long term blood sugar (HbA1c; %) in male type 2 diabetics before and after 10 weeks of either 10-20-30 training (10-20-30) and moderate intensity continuous training (moderate intensity). Note that only the group doing 10-20-30 training had a marked decrease in long term blood sugar.

Effect of 10-20-30 training on body composition of diabetes patients

The diabetes patients conducting the 10-20-30 training had a 4%-fall in fat mass from 35.3 to 33.9 kg, with a corresponding decrease in fat percentage of 4% (see Figure 14). These changes were similar to those observed (4% and 3%, respectively) in the diabetes group doing the moderate intensity work. Apparently, the 10-20-30 training had the same positive effects on body composition as moderate intensity training, although the training volume was less that the half.

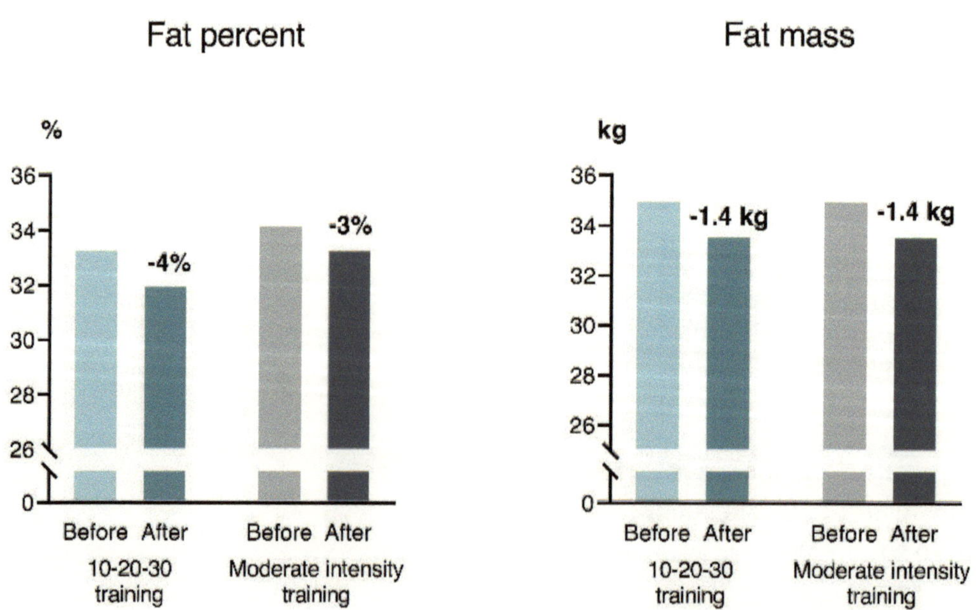

Figure 14. Fat percentage (%) (left) and fat mass (kg) (right) in male type 2 diabetics before and after 10 weeks of either 10-20-30 training (10-20-30) or moderate intensity continuous training (moderate intensity). Note that both groups decreased fat percentage and mass significantly.

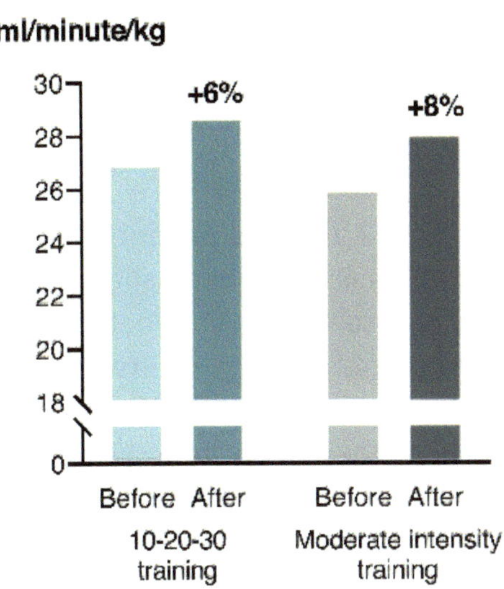

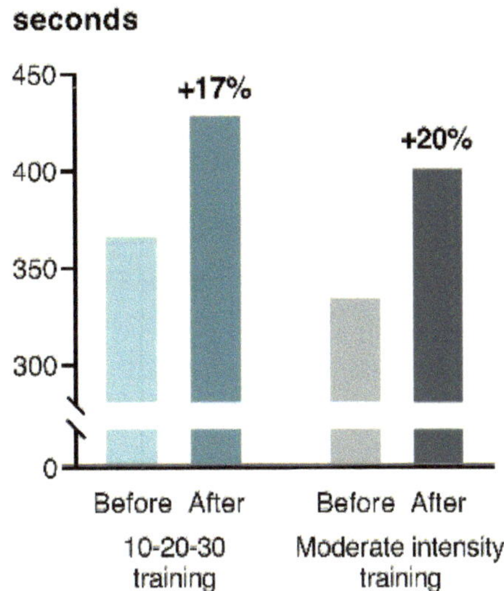

Figure 15. Maximum oxygen uptake (left) and performance (right) in male type 2 diabetics before and after 10 weeks of either 10-20-30 training (10-20-30) or moderate intensity continuous training (moderate intensity). Note that the two groups had the same improvements.

Effect of 10-20-30 training on maximum oxygen uptake and performance of diabetes patients

In the 10-20-30 training group maximum oxygen uptake increased by 7%, and by 8% in the moderate intensity training group (see Figure 15). Performance during an incremental test increased 17% in the 10-20-30 training group and by 20% in the moderate intensity training group (see Figure 15).

Perspectives for diabetes patients

Type 2 diabetes is associated with an inactive lifestyle and obesity. The adherence to exercise training within these patients is lower than in healthy people. However, in the study the compliance was >83% for both training groups, and no injuries occurred, suggesting that it is easy to implement 10-20-30 training for patients with type 2 diabetes.

10-20-30 training was superior in lowering long term blood sugar than moderate-intensity training, and the ~0.5% point reduction in HbA_{1c} in the study did, among other things, reduce the risk of diabetes related death by ~10%. It was also shown to reduce fat mass, increase maximum oxygen uptake and improve performance. Thus, the 10-20-30 training is of great relevance and can be implement in the society as an effective and time efficient treatment and prevention of Type 2 diabetes.

10-20-30 training programme for diabetes patients

Table 10 presents a 10-20-30 cycle training program for type 2 diabetes patients. The loading is progressively increasing and the load during the 10-second period should only be slightly higher than the 20-second periods in the first weeks (see number of loading in Table 10). In the first three weeks the number of training sessions is two, where after the patient is doing three sessions per week. One of the sessions could be in the weekend, but the training can also be conducted on two/three week days, they just have to be separated by one day of recovery. In the first weeks the training lasts 10-20 minutes, then 20-30 minutes. If you miss a training session one week, it is not a problem, just make sure you are completing all the sessions in the following week.

The program shows the loading for the 30- (blue), 20- (green) and 10- (red) second periods. As you get in better shape, the loading within the various categories will increase. The program does also provide suggestions of when to test your selves.

The loading is relative and given as:

	Load
1	No load
2	Low load
3	Low/moderate load
4	Moderate load
5	Moderate/high load
6	High load

Table 10. A 10-20-30 training program for diabetes patients.

*Week	First session Monday/Tuesday/ Wednesday	Second session Wednesday/Thursday/ Friday	Third session Saturday/ Sunday	Intensity# 30 20 10
Week 1	5 min warm-up 1x5min 10-20-30	5 min warm-up 2x5min 10-20-30 Recovery 4 min		1 2 4 1 2 4
Week 2	5 min warm-up 2x5min 10-20-30 Recovery 4 min	5 min warm-up 2x5min 10-20-30 Recovery 4 min		1 2 4 1 2 4
Week 3	5 min warm-up 2x5min 10-20-30 Recovery 3 min	5 min warm-up 2x5min 10-20-30 Recovery 3 min		1 2 5 1 2 5
Week 4	5 min warm-up 2x5min 10-20-30 Recovery 3 min	5 min warm-up 2x5min 10-20-30 Recovery 3 min	5 min warm-up 2x5min 10-20-30 Recovery 3 min	1 2 5 1 2 5 1 2 5
Week 5	5 min warm-up 2x5min 10-20-30 Recovery 3 min	5 min warm-up 3x5min 10-20-30 Recovery 4 min	5 min warm-up 2x5min 10-20-30 Recovery 3 min	1 3 5 1 2 5 1 3 5
Week 6	Test (6 min) and 1x5 min 10-20-30	5 min warm-up 3x5min 10-20-30 Recovery 4 min	5 min warm-up 2x5min 10-20-30 Recovery 3 min	1 3 5 1 3 5 2 3 5
Week 7	5 min warm-up 3x5min 10-20-30 Recovery 4 min	5 min warm-up 2x5min 10-20-30 Recovery 3 min	5 min warm-up 3x5min 10-20-30 Recovery 4 min	2 3 5 2 4 5 2 3 5
Week 8	5 min warm-up 3x5min 10-20-30 Recovery 4 min	5 min warm-up 2x5min 10-20-30 Recovery 3 min	5 min warm-up 3x5min 10-20-30 Recovery 4 min	2 3 5 2 4 5 2 3 5

Week 9	5 min warm-up	5 min warm-up	5 min warm-up	2	3	5
	3x5min 10-20-30	2x5min 10-20-30	3x5min 10-20-30	2	4	5
	Recovery 4 min	Recovery 3 min	Recovery 4 min	2	3	5
Week 10	5 min warm-up	5 min warm-up	5 min warm-up	2	4	5
	3x5min 10-20-30	2x5min 10-20-30	3x5min 10-20-30	2	4	5
	Recovery 4 min	Recovery 3 min	Recovery 3 min	2	4	5
Week 11	Test (6 min) and	5 min warm-up	5 min warm-up	2	4	5
	2x5 min 10-20-30	3x5min 10-20-30	3x5min 10-20-30	2	4	5
	Recovery 3 min	Recovery 3 min	Recovery 3 min	2	4	5
Week 12	5 min warm-up	5 min warm-up	5 min warm-up	2	4	5
	3x5min 10-20-30	3x5min 10-20-30	3x5min 10-20-30	2	4	6
	Recovery 3 min	Recovery 4 min	Recovery 3 min	2	4	5
Week 13	5 min warm-up	5 min warm-up	5 min warm-up	2	4	6
	3x5min 10-20-30	3x5min 10-20-30	3x5min 10-20-30	2	4	5
	Recovery 3 min	Recovery 2 min	Recovery 3 min	2	4	6
Week 14	5 min warm-up	5 min warm-up	5 min warm-up	2	4	6
	3x5min 10-20-30	3x5min 10-20-30	3x5min 10-20-30	2	4	5
	Recovery 3 min	Recovery 2 min	Recovery 3 min	2	4	6
Week 15	5 min warm-up	5 min warm-up	5 min warm-up	2	4	6
	3x5min 10-20-30	3x5min 10-20-30	3x5min 10-20-30	2	4	6
	Recovery 3 min	Recovery 3 min	Recovery 3 min	2	4	6
Week 16	Test (6 min) and	5 min warm-up	5 min warm-up	2	4	6
	2x5 min 10-20-30	3x5min 10-20-30	3x5min 10-20-30	2	4	6
	Recovery 3 min	Recovery 2 min	Recovery 2 min	2	4	6
Week 17	5 min warm-up	5 min warm-up	5 min warm-up	2	4	6
	3x5min 10-20-30	3x5min 10-20-30	3x5min 10-20-30	2	4	6
	Recovery 2 min	Recovery 2 min	Recovery 2 min	2	4	6
Week 18	5 min warm-up	5 min warm-up	5 min warm-up	2	4	6
	3x5min 10-20-30	3x5min 10-20-30	3x5min 10-20-30	2	4	6

	Recovery 2 min	Recovery 2 min	Recovery 2 min	2 4 6
Week 19	5 min warm-up	5 min warm-up	5 min warm-up	2 4 6
	3x5min 10-20-30	3x5min 10-20-30	3x5min 10-20-30	2 4 6
	Recovery 2 min	Recovery 2 min	Recovery 2 min	2 4 6
Week 20	5 min warm-up	5 min warm-up	5 min warm-up	2 4 6
	3x5min 10-20-30	3x5min 10-20-30	3x5min 10-20-30	2 4 6
	Recovery 2 min	Recovery 2 min	Recovery 2 min	2 4 6
Week 21	Test (6 min) and	5 min warm-up	5 min warm-up	2 4 6
	2x5 min 10-20-30	3x5min 10-20-30	3x5min 10-20-30	2 4 6
	Recovery 2 min	Recovery 2 min	Recovery 2 min	2 4 6
	Continue the program from week 20			

* Enter the weeks according to when you start the training period.

Hypertensive

Hypertension, also known as high blood pressure, is a medical condition in which the blood pressure in the arteries is persistently elevated. About 90–95% of cases are primary, defined as high blood pressure due to nonspecific lifestyle and genetic factors. It is associated with impairments in cardiovascular structure and function, and is a well-established risk factor for developing cardiovascular diseases. More than 20% of the population globally are hypertensive, and hypertension is believed to be a factor in about 20% of all deaths.

Regular physical activity can lower blood pressure and decrease the risk of health complications.

10-20-30 training of hypertensive

In a study, untrained individuals aged 55-65 years with hypertension and age-matched normotensive controls conducted 6 weeks of 10-20-30 training. The training was conducted on cycle ergometers. Both groups did 10-20-30 training consisting of five consecutive 1-minute intervals divided into 30-, 20-, and 10-second intervals at an intensity corresponding to ~30%, ~50% and ~100% of maximal intensity, respectively. For the first two weeks of training two 5-minute bouts, interspersed by 3 min of recovery, were conducted. The last four weeks the subjects had three 5-minute bouts per training session interspersed by 3 min of recovery, and the number of weekly training sessions was increased from 2 to 3.

The participants completed 98% of the training sessions. Heart rate during the training sessions was similar in the two groups with about 60% of the time spent between 80-90% of maximum heart rate and 13% above 90 % of maximum heart rate.

Effect of 10-20-30 training on blood pressure for hypertensive

In the hypertensive group systolic blood pressure (for explanation see page 32) decreased by 9 mmHg with 10-20-30 training, whereas diastolic blood pressure decreased by 5 mmHg (see Figure 16; see page 74). These changes can be compared to decrease in systolic and diastolic blood pressure by 4 and 2 mmHg, respectively, typically observed after a 12-week programme of moderate intensity exercise for 30-60 minutes three times a week. The reduction in systolic blood pressure of 9 mmHg with the 10-20-30 training is of great clinical relevance as a decrease of 10 mmHg in systolic blood pressure is associated with ~40 % lower risk of stroke death and ~30 % lower risk of death from ischemic heart disease. The normotensive group had a decrease in systolic and diastolic blood pressure of 5 and 3 mmHg, respectively, with the 10-20-30 training (see Figure 16).

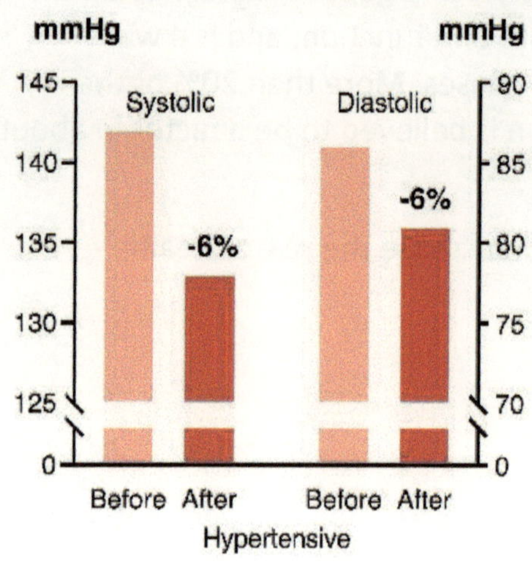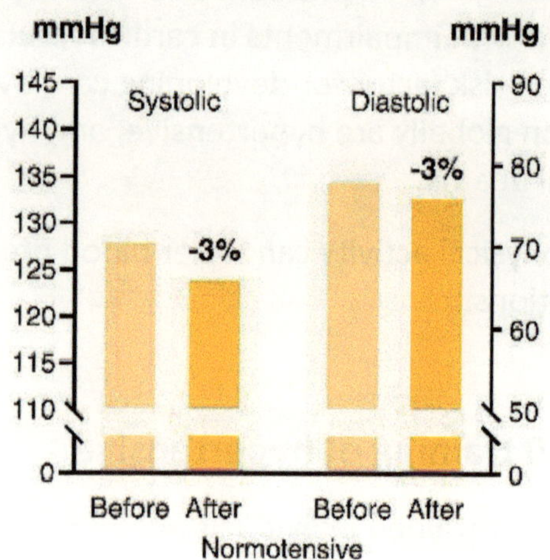

Figure 16. Systolic and diastolic blood pressure for hypertensive (left) and normotensive (right) before and after a 6-week period of 10-20-30 training. Note that the hypertensive group had an amazing decrease in systolic blood pressure, and also in diastolic blood pressure.

Effect of 10-20-30 training on body composition

Fat mass decreased with the six weeks of 10-20-30 training from 29.5 to 27.9 kg in the hypertensive group and from 27.7 to 26.1 kg in the normotensive group (see Figure 17). Similarly, the decrease in fat percentage was from 33.1% to 31.4% and 33.1% to 31.7%, respectively. Also visceral fat decreased in both groups (see Figure 17), whereas fat free mass improved from 59.1 to 60.1 kg in the hypertensive group and did not change in the normotensive group (56.2 vs. 56.4 kg).

Effect of 10-20-30 training on maximum oxygen uptake and performance of hypertensive

Maximum oxygen uptake improved by 3% and 8% with 10-20-30 training in the hypertensive and normotensive group, respectively, and performance during an incremental test on a cycle increased by 7% and 12%, respectively (see Figure 18).

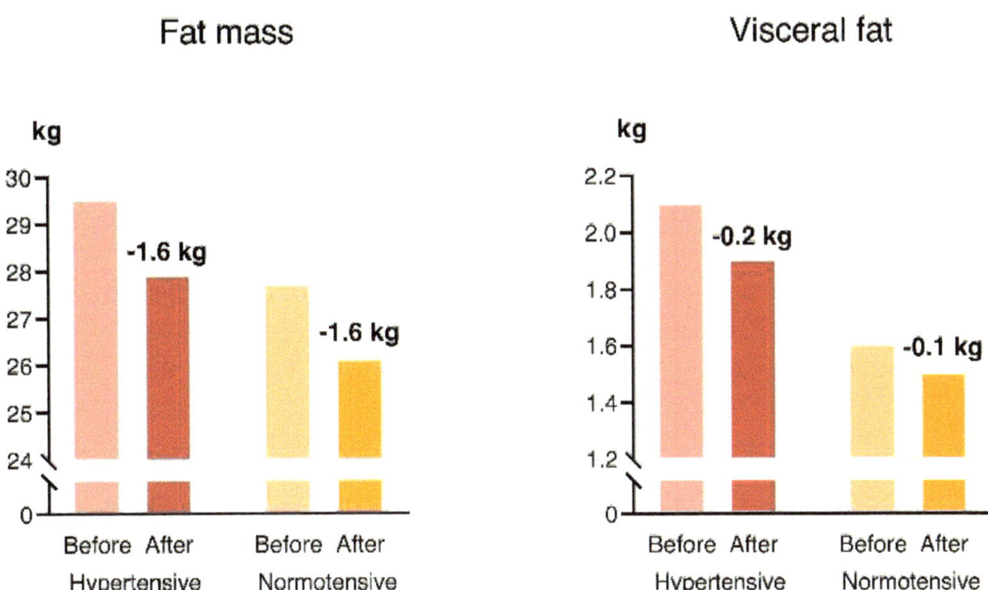

Figure 17. Fat mass (left) and visceral fat (right) for hypertensive and normotensive before and after a 6-week period of 10-20-30 training. Note that both groups had marked decrease in fat mass and also a decrease in the amount of visceral fat.

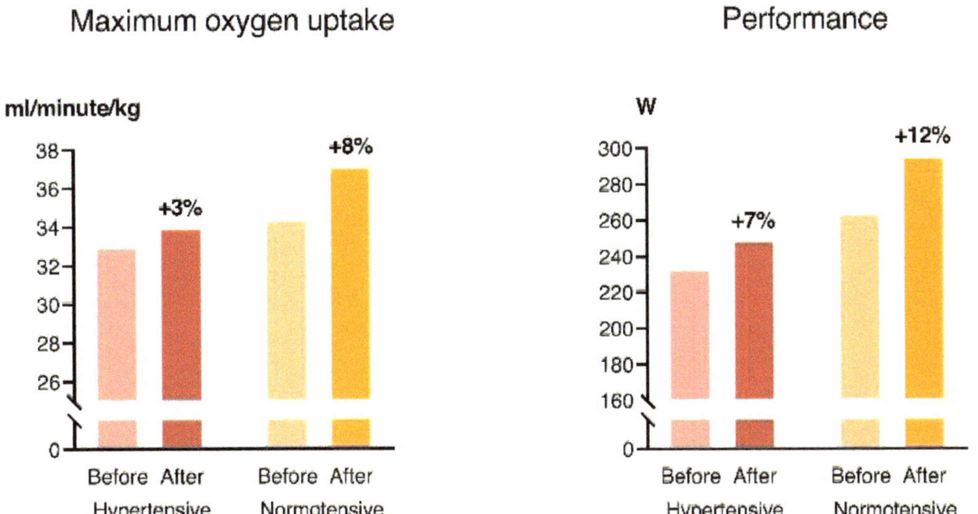

Figure 18. Maximum oxygen uptake (right) and performance (left) for hypertensive and normotensive before and after a 6-week period of 10-20-30 training. Note that both groups had a marked increase in maximum oxygen uptake and performance.

Perspectives of 10-20-30 training for hypertensive

The reduction in systolic and diastolic blood pressure of 9/5 mmHg with 10-20-30 training in the hypertensive subjects is of great importance and does decrease the risk of death from a stroke or from ischemic heart disease with more than 30 %. The observed increase in maximum oxygen uptake of 2 ml per minute per kg in the hypertensive group is also of clinical relevance, as each 1 ml per minute per kg increase in maximum oxygen uptake has been shown to be associated with a 45-day increase in longevity. In addition, the loos of about 1.5 kg of fat, and particular visceral fat, reduced the risk of metabolic diseases significantly. Thus, the 10-20-30 training only conducted for 6 weeks was very efficient in improving the health conditions for both the hypertensive and the normotensive participants.

10-20-30 training program for hypertensive

Table 11 (see page 78) presents a 10-20-30 training program for hypertensive. The loading is progressively increasing and the load during the 10-second period should only be slightly higher than the 20-second periods in the first weeks (see number of loading in the table). In the first three weeks the number of training sessions is two, where after the hypertensive is doing three sessions per week. One of the sessions could be in the weekend, but the training can also be conducted on two/three week days, they just have to be separated by a day of recover. In the first weeks the training lasts 10-20 minutes, then 20-30 minutes. If you miss a training session one week, it is not a problem, just make sure you are completing all the sessions in the following week.

The programme shows the loading for the 30- (blue), 20- (green) and 10- (red) second periods. As you get in better shape, the loading within the various categories will increase. The programme does also provide suggestions of when to test your selves.

The loading is relative and given as:

	Load
1	No load
2	Low load
3	Low/moderate load
4	Moderate load
5	Moderate/high load
6	High load

Table 11. A 10-20-30 training program for hypertensive.

*Week	First session Monday/Tuesday/ Wednesday	Second session Wednesday/Thursday/ Friday	Third session Saturday/ Sunday	Intensity# 30 20 10
Week 1	5 min warm-up 1x5min 10-20-30	5 min warm-up 2x5min 10-20-30 Recovery 3 min		1 2 4 1 2 4
Week 2	5 min warm-up 2x5min 10-20-30 Recovery 3 min	5 min warm-up 2x5min 10-20-30 Recovery 3 min		1 2 4 1 2 4
Week 3	5 min warm-up 3x5min 10-20-30 Recovery 3 min	5 min warm-up 3x5min 10-20-30 Recovery 3 min		1 2 4 1 2 4
Week 4	5 min warm-up 3x5min 10-20-30 Recovery 3 min	5 min warm-up 3x5min 10-20-30 Recovery 3 min	5 min warm-up 3x5min 10-20-30 Recovery 3 min	1 2 5 1 2 5 1 2 5
Week 5	5 min warm-up 3x5min 10-20-30 Recovery 3 min	5 min warm-up 3x5min 10-20-30 Recovery 4 min	5 min warm-up 3x5min 10-20-30 Recovery 3 min	1 2 5 1 2 5 1 2 5
Week 6	Test (6 min) and 1x5 min 10-20-30	5 min warm-up 3x5min 10-20-30 Recovery 3 min	5 min warm-up 3x5min 10-20-30 Recovery 3 min	1 3 5 1 3 5 1 3 5
Week 7	5 min warm-up 3x5min 10-20-30 Recovery 3 min	5 min warm-up 2x5min 10-20-30 Recovery 3 min	5 min warm-up 3x5min 10-20-30 Recovery 3 min	2 3 5 2 3 5 2 3 5

Week 8	5 min warm-up	5 min warm-up	5 min warm-up	2	3	5
	3x5min 10-20-30	3x5min 10-20-30	3x5min 10-20-30	2	4	5
	Recovery 3 min	Recovery 3 min	Recovery 3 min	2	4	5
Week 9	5 min warm-up	5 min warm-up	5 min warm-up	2	4	5
	3x5min 10-20-30	3x5min 10-20-30	3x5min 10-20-30	2	4	5
	Recovery 3 min	Recovery 3 min	Recovery 3 min	2	4	5
Week 10	5 min warm-up	5 min warm-up	5 min warm-up	2	4	6
	3x5min 10-20-30	2x5min 10-20-30	3x5min 10-20-30	2	4	6
	Recovery 4 min	Recovery 4 min	Recovery 4 min	2	4	6
Week 11	Test (6 min) and	5 min warm-up	5 min warm-up	2	4	6
	2x5 min 10-20-30	3x5min 10-20-30	3x5min 10-20-30	2	4	6
	Recovery 3 min	Recovery 3 min	Recovery 3 min	2	4	6
Week 12	5 min warm-up	5 min warm-up	5 min warm-up	2	4	6
	3x5min 10-20-30	3x5min 10-20-30	3x5min 10-20-30	2	4	6
	Recovery 3 min	Recovery 3 min	Recovery 3 min	2	4	6
Week 13	5 min warm-up	5 min warm-up	5 min warm-up	2	4	6
	3x5min 10-20-30	3x5min 10-20-30	3x5min 10-20-30	2	4	6
	3 min	Recovery 3 min	Recovery 3 min	2	4	6
Week 14	5 min warm-up	5 min warm-up	5 min warm-up	2	4	6
	3x5min 10-20-30	3x5min 10-20-30	3x5min 10-20-30	2	4	6
	Recovery 3 min	Recovery 3 min	Recovery 3 min	2	4	6
Week 15	5 min warm-up	5 min warm-up	5 min warm-up	2	4	6
	3x5min 10-20-30	3x5min 10-20-30	3x5min 10-20-30	2	4	6
	Recovery 3 min	Recovery 3 min	Recovery 3 min	2	4	6
Week 16	Test (6 min) and	5 min warm-up	5 min warm-up	2	4	6
	2x5 min 10-20-30	4x5min 10-20-30	4x5min 10-20-30	2	4	6
	Recovery 3 min	Recovery 4 min	Recovery 4 min	2	4	6
Week 17	5 min warm-up	5 min warm-up	5 min warm-up	2	4	6
	4x5min 10-20-30	4x5min 10-20-30	4x5min 10-20-30	2	4	6

				2 4 6
	Recovery 3 min	Recovery 3 min	Recovery 3 min	2 4 6
Week 18	5 min warm-up	5 min warm-up	5 min warm-up	2 4 6
	4x5min 10-20-30	4x5min 10-20-30	4x5min 10-20-30	2 4 6
	Recovery 3 min	Recovery 3 min	Recovery 3 min	2 4 6
Week 19	5 min warm-up	5 min warm-up	5 min warm-up	2 4 6
	4x5min 10-20-30	4x5min 10-20-30	4x5min 10-20-30	2 4 6
	Recovery 3 min	Recovery 3 min	Recovery 3 min	2 4 6
Week 20	5 min warm-up	5 min warm-up	5 min warm-up	2 4 6
	4x5min 10-20-30	4x5min 10-20-30	4x5min 10-20-30	2 4 6
	Recovery 2 min	Recovery 2 min	Recovery 2 min	2 4 6
Week 21	Test (6 min) and	5 min warm-up	5 min warm-up	2 4 6
	2x5 min 10-20-30	4x5min 10-20-30	4x5min 10-20-30	2 4 6
	Recovery 2 min	Recovery 2 min	Recovery 2 min	2 4 6
	Continue the program from week 20			

* Enter the weeks according to when you start the training period

Asthma patients

Asthma is a common long-term inflammatory disease of the airways of the lungs. It is characterized by variable and recurring symptoms, reversible airflow obstruction, and easily triggered bronchospasms. Symptoms include episodes of wheezing, coughing, chest tightness, and shortness of breath. These may occur a few times a day or a few times per week. Depending on the person, asthma symptoms may become worse at night or with exercise. More than 350 million people globally have asthma. It has been estimated to cause about 400,000 deaths annually, most of which occur in the developing world. Asthma is thought to be caused by a combination of genetic and environmental factors, including exposure to air pollution and allergens.

Training has been found to improve asthma control, airway hyperresponsiveness and airway inflammation. However, engaging in physical activity can be a challenge for patients with asthma, since many experience exercise-induced asthma symptoms. This may cause them to avoid physical activity, leading to deconditioning and poor cardiorespiratory fitness. High-intensity interval training is today widely practiced because of its superior efficacy to improve exercise capacity when compared to low- to moderate-intensity training, and 10-20-30 training has been shown to be feasible for asthma patients and improve their control of asthma.

10-20-30 training of asthma patients

In a study female and male asthma patients, aged 18-65 years, were divided into a training group, a diet group, a training and diet group and a control group, which maintained usual physical activity levels and diet.

The training groups conducted 8 weeks of 10-20-30 training indoor on bikes 3 times a week, supervised by an instructor. Each session included 10 minutes of warming-up at a low intensity followed by two 5-min intervals the first two weeks, three 5-min intervals the next three weeks and four 5-min intervals the last three weeks. Each 5-minute interval consisted of five consecutive 1-minutes intervals with 30, 20, and 10 seconds at an intensity corresponding to <30%, <60% and >90% of maximal intensity, respectively. Patients took two puffs of their regular short acting beta-2 agonist 10-15 minutes prior to the training and during the training sessions, if necessary to prevent bronchoconstriction. The patients were able to maintain the very high intensity during the training sessions without getting asthma symptoms that could not be relieved with 1-2 puffs of beta-2 agonist or a short pause (1–2 minutes) from training. The time spent between 90 and 100% of maximum heart rate during training was 6 minutes during the first 2 weeks, 9 minutes during the following 3 weeks, and 11 minutes during the last 3 weeks. The training was conducted in a hospital setting, and the training groups completed 90% of the planned training sessions

The patients in the two diet groups prepared their own food with a high protein content (25–30% of energy) and with low glycemic index carbohydrates (<55%), i.e. carbohydrates which does only increase blood sugar slightly, as well as a minimum of 300 grams of vegetables plus two pieces of fruit per day.

Effect of 10-20-30 training and diet on asthma control and quality of life for asthma patients

Both training groups and the diet group improved their control of asthma (see Figure 19) and when asked about asthma related quality of life all four groups improved, with the training and diet group having the greatest improvement (see Figure 20).

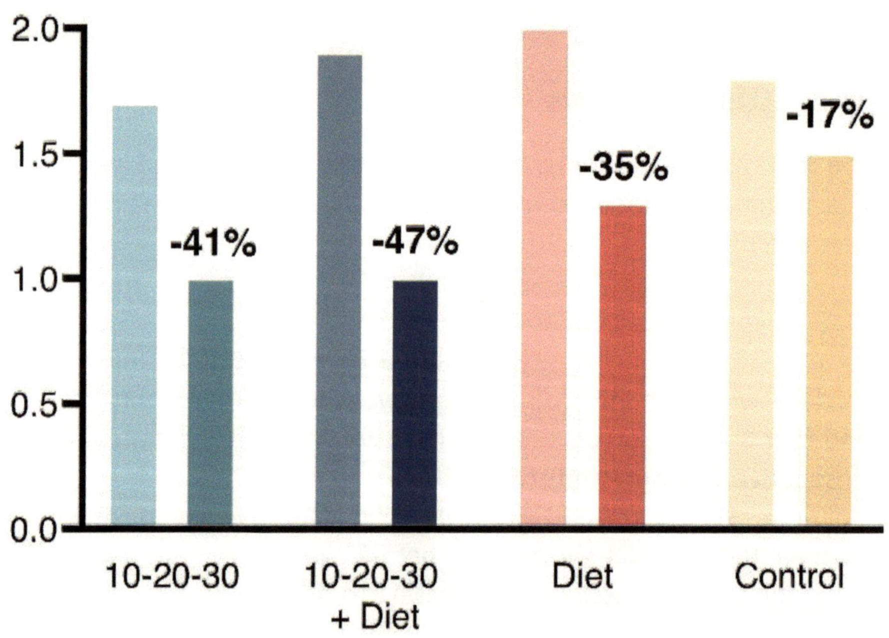

Figure 19. Control of asthma (relative values - lower value better control) for asthma patients before and after an 8-week period with 10-20-30 training (10-20-30), 10-20-30 training and diet intervention (10-20-30 + Diet), diet intervention (Diet) and no intervention (Control). Note that the training and diet groups improved significantly.

Asthma related quality of life

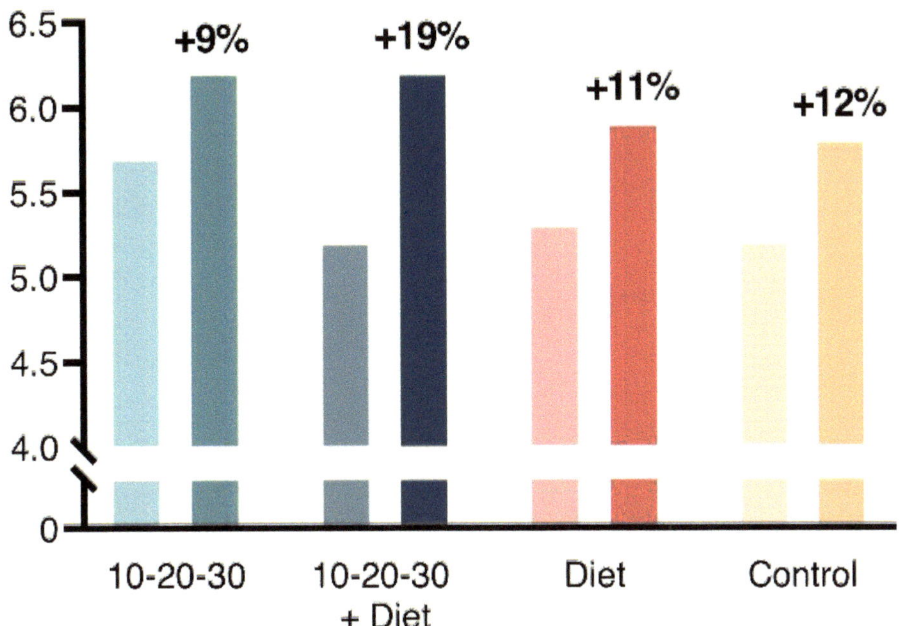

Figure 20. Asthma related quality of life (relative values - higher value better quality) for asthma patients before and after an 8-week period with 10-20-30 training (10-20-30), 10-20-30 training and diet intervention (10-20-30 + Diet), diet intervention (Diet) and no intervention (Control). Note that the training and diet group had the largest improvement.

Effect of 10-20-30 training and diet on body composition in asthma patients

The training groups and the diet group lowered the body weight and fat mass with the intervention (see Figure 21). For example, the 10-20-30 training and diet group reduced fat mass by an amazing 3.9 kg.

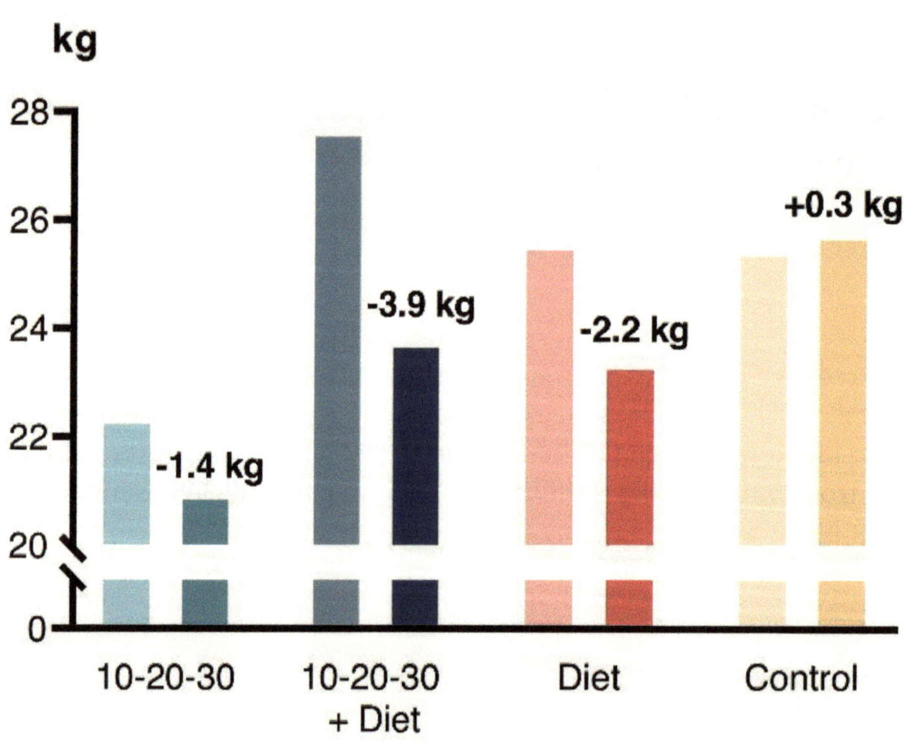

Figure 21. Fat mass for asthma patients before bod after an 8-week period with 10-20-30 training (10-20-30), 10-20-30 training and diet intervention (10-20-30 + Diet), diet intervention (Diet) and no intervention (Control). Note the marked decrease in fat mass for the training and diet groups.

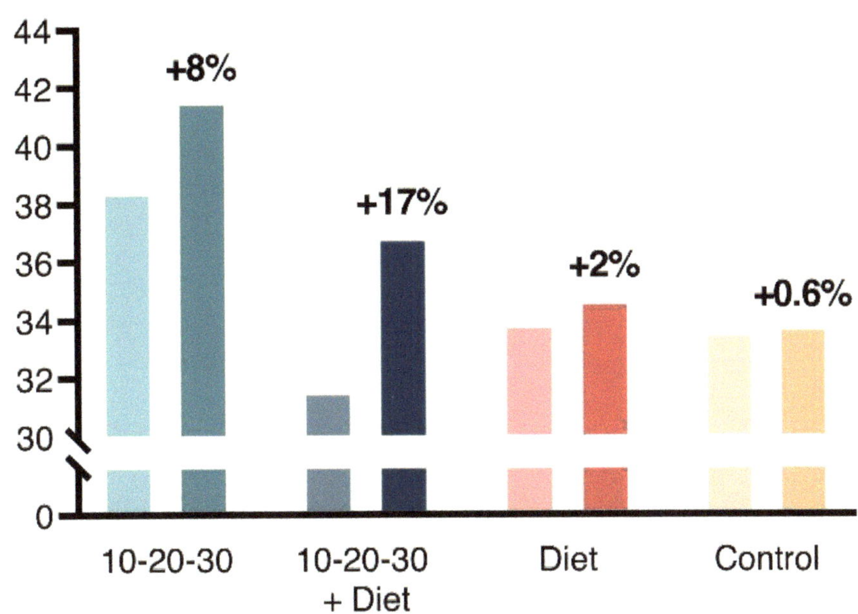

Figure 22. Maximum oxygen uptake for asthma patients before and after an 8-week period with 10-20-30 training (10-20-30), 10-20-30 training and diet intervention (10-20-30 + D), diet intervention (Diet) and no intervention (Control). Note that only the training groups had significant improvements in maximum oxygen uptake.

Effect of 10-20-30 training and diet on maximum oxygen uptake and performance of asthma patients

Maximum oxygen uptake increased from 38.4 to 41.5 ml/kg/min in the training group and from 31.5 to 36.8 ml/kg/min in the training and diet group (see Figure 22), whereas the diet and control group did not have any change.

Perspectives of 10-20-30 training for asthma patients

The study showed that it is feasible and time efficient to conduct 10-20-30 training with asthma patients, which is an advantage in a busy modern lifestyle, where lack of time can be a barrier to attend training.

10-20-30 training program for asthma patients

Table 12 presents a 10-20-30 training program for asthma patients. The loading is progressively increasing and the load during the 10-second period should only be slightly higher than the 20-second periods in the first weeks (see number of loading in Table 12). If you feel breathless, you may take 1-2 puff of your medicine. In the first three weeks the number of training sessions is two, where after you are doing three sessions per week. One of the sessions could be in the weekend, but the training can also be conducted on two/three week days, they just have to be separated by a day of recovery. In the first weeks the training lasts 10-20 minutes, then 20-30 minutes. If you miss a training session one week, it is not a problem, just make sure you are completing all the sessions in the following week.

The program shows the loading for the 30- (blue), 20- (green) and 10- (red) seconds periods. As you get in better shape, the loading within the various categories will increase. The program does also provide suggestions of when to test your selves.

The loading is relative and given as:

	Load
1	No load
2	Low load
3	Low/moderate load
4	Moderate load
5	Moderate/high load
6	High load

Table 12. A 10-20-30 training program for asthma patients.

*Week	First session Monday/Tuesday/ Wednesday	Second session Wednesday/Thursday/ Friday	Third session Saturday/ Sunday	Intensity# 30 20 10
Week 1	5 min warm-up 1x5min 10-20-30	5 min warm-up 2x5min 10-20-30 Recovery 4 min		1 2 4 1 2 4
Week 2	5 min warm-up 2x5min 10-20-30 Recovery 4 min	5 min warm-up 2x5min 10-20-30 Recovery 4 min		1 2 4 1 2 4
Week 3	5 min warm-up 3x5min 10-20-30 Recovery 4 min	5 min warm-up 3x5min 10-20-30 Recovery 4 min		1 2 4 1 2 4
Week 4	5 min warm-up 3x5min 10-20-30 Recovery 4 min	5 min warm-up 3x5min 10-20-30 Recovery 4 min	5 min warm-up 3x5min 10-20-30 Recovery 4 min	1 2 4 1 2 5 1 2 5
Week 5	5 min warm-up 3x5min 10-20-30 Recovery 4 min	5 min warm-up 3x5min 10-20-30 Recovery 4 min	5 min warm-up 3x5min 10-20-30 Recovery 4 min	1 3 5 1 3 5 1 3 5
Week 6	Test (6 min) and 1x5 min 10-20-30	5 min warm-up 3x5min 10-20-30 Recovery 4 min	5 min warm-up 3x5min 10-20-30 Recovery 4 min	1 3 5 1 3 5 1 3 5
Week 7	5 min warm-up 3x5min 10-20-30 Recovery 4 min	5 min warm-up 3x5min 10-20-30 Recovery 4 min	5 min warm-up 3x5min 10-20-30 Recovery 4 min	2 3 5 2 3 5 2 3 5
Week 8	5 min warm-up 3x5min 10-20-30	5 min warm-up 3x5min 10-20-30	5 min warm-up 3x5min 10-20-30	2 4 5 2 4 5

	Recovery 4 min	Recovery 4 min	Recovery 4 min	2	4	5
Week 9	5 min warm-up	5 min warm-up	5 min warm-up	2	4	5
	3x5min 10-20-30	2x5min 10-20-30	3x5min 10-20-30	2	4	5
	Recovery 3 min	Recovery 3 min	Recovery 3 min	2	4	5
Week 10	5 min warm-up	5 min warm-up	5 min warm-up	2	4	5
	3x5min 10-20-30	3x5min 10-20-30	3x5min 10-20-30	2	4	5
	Recovery 3 min	Recovery 3 min	Recovery 3 min	2	4	5
Week 11	Test (6 min) and	5 min warm-up	5 min warm-up	2	4	5
	2x5 min 10-20-30	3x5min 10-20-30	4x5min 10-20-30	2	4	5
	Recovery 3 min	Recovery 3 min	Recovery 3 min	2	4	5
Week 12	5 min warm-up	5 min warm-up	5 min warm-up	2	4	5
	4x5min 10-20-30	4x5min 10-20-30	4x5min 10-20-30	2	4	5
	Recovery 3 min	Recovery 3 min	Recovery 3 min	2	4	5
Week 13	5 min warm-up	5 min warm-up	5 min warm-up	2	4	5
	4x5min 10-20-30	4x5min 10-20-30	3x5min 10-20-30	2	4	5
	Recovery 3 min	Recovery 3 min	Recovery 3 min	2	4	5
Week 14	5 min warm-up	5 min warm-up	5 min warm-up	2	4	6
	4x5min 10-20-30	4x5min 10-20-30	4x5min 10-20-30	2	4	6
	Recovery 3 min	Recovery 3 min	Recovery 3 min	2	4	6
Week 15	5 min warm-up	5 min warm-up	5 min warm-up	2	4	6
	4x5min 10-20-30	4x5min 10-20-30	4x5min 10-20-30	2	4	6
	Recovery 3 min	Recovery 3 min	Recovery 3 min	2	4	6
Week 16	Test (6 min) and	5 min warm-up	5 min warm-up	2	4	6
	2x5 min 10-20-30	4x5min 10-20-30	4x5min 10-20-30	2	4	6
	Recovery 3 min	Recovery 3 min	Recovery 3 min	2	4	6
Week 17	5 min warm-up	5 min warm-up	5 min warm-up	2	4	6
	4x5min 10-20-30	4x5min 10-20-30	4x5min 10-20-30	2	4	6
	Recovery 2 min	Recovery 2 min	Recovery 2 min	2	4	6
Week 18	5 min warm-up	5 min warm-up	5 min warm-up	2	4	6

				2	4	6
	4x5min 10-20-30	4x5min 10-20-30	4x5min 10-20-30	2	4	6
	Recovery 2 min	Recovery 2 min	Recovery 2 min	2	4	6
Week 19	5 min warm-up	5 min warm-up	5 min warm-up	2	4	6
	4x5min 10-20-30	4x5min 10-20-30	4x5min 10-20-30	2	4	6
	Recovery 2 min	Recovery 2 min	Recovery 2 min	2	4	6
Week 20	5 min warm-up	5 min warm-up	5 min warm-up	2	4	6
	4x5min 10-20-30	4x5min 10-20-30	4x5min 10-20-30	2	4	6
	Recovery 2 min	Recovery 2 min	Recovery 2 min	2	4	6
Week 21	Test (6 min) and	5 min warm-up	5 min warm-up	2	4	6
	2x5 min 10-20-30	4x5min 10-20-30	4x5min 10-20-30	2	4	6
	Recovery 2 min	Recovery 2 min	Recovery 2 min	2	4	6
	Continue the program from week 20					

* Enter the weeks according to when you start the training period.

Synopsis

10-20-30 training has in scientific studies been shown to be very effective to improve performance and health, even for well-trained who can reduce the volume of training and make significant improvements. The 10-20-30 training is also feasible for various patients groups, such as hypertensive, diabetic and asthma patients, and more effective than traditional moderate intensity training of much longer duration. Actually, that 10-20-30 training can be completed in a short time is another great advantage, and makes it useful in a busy schedule.

References and further reading

Baasch-Skytte T, Lemgart CT, Oehlenschläger MH, Petersen PE, Hostrup M, Bangsbo J, Gunnarsson TP (2020). Efficacy of 10-20-30 training versus moderate-intensity continuous training on HbA1c, body composition and maximum oxygen uptake in male patients with type 2 diabetes: A randomized controlled trial. Diabetes Obes Metab 22: 767-778.

Bangsbo J, Gunnarsson TP, Wendell J, Nybo L, Thomassen M (2009). Reduced volume and increased training intensity elevate muscle Na+-K+ pump alpha2-subunit expression as well as short- and long-term work capacity in humans. J Appl Physiol 107: 1771-1780.

Bangsbo J (2015). Performance in sports - with specific emphasis on the effect of intensified training. Scand J Med Sci Sports 25: 88-99.

Faelli E, Ferrando V, Bisio A, Ferrando M, La Torre A, Panasci M, Ruggeri P (2019). Effects of two high-intensity interval training concepts in recreational runners. Int J Sports Med 40: 639-644.

Fiorenza M, Gunnarsson TP, Ehlers TS, Bangsbo J (2019). High-intensity exercise training ameliorates aberrant expression of markers of mitochondrial turnover but not oxidative damage in skeletal muscle of men with essential hypertension. Acta Phys 225: e13208.

Gliemann L, Gunnarsson TP, Hellsten Y, Bangsbo J (2015). 10-20-30 training increases performance and lowers blood pressure and VEGF in runners. Scand J Med Sci Sport 25: 479-489.

Gunnarsson TP, Bangsbo J (2012). The 10-20-30 training concept improves performance and health profile in moderately trained runners. J Appl Physiol 113:16-24.

Gunnarsson TP, Ehlers TS, Fiorenza MT, Nyberg M, Bangsbo J (2020). Essential hypertension is associated with impaired smooth muscle cell vasodilator responsiveness that is reversed by high-intensity exercise training. Am J Physiol, Cell Physiol 318: C1252-C1263.

Hostrup M, Gunnarsson TP, Fiorenza M, Mørch K, Onslev J, Pedersen KM, Bangsbo J (2019). In-season adaptations to intense intermittent training and sprint interval training in sub-elite football players. Scand J Med Sci Sports 29: 669-677.

Iaia FM, Bangsbo J (2010). Speed endurance training is a powerful stimulus for physiological adaptations and performance improvements of athletes. Scand J Med Sci Sports, Suppl 2: 11-23.

Pedersen BK, Saltin B (2006). Evidence for prescribing exercise as therapy in chronic disease. Scand J Med Sci Sports, Suppl 1: 3-63.

Skovgaard C, Christiansen D, Rodriguez AM, Bangsbo J. Similar improvements in 5-km performance and maximal oxygen uptake with sub-maximal and maximal 10-20-30 training in runners, but increase in muscle oxidative phosphorylation occur only with maximal effort training. Scand J Med Sci Sports, in press.

Toennesen LL, Meteran H, Hostrup M, Wium Geiker NR, Jensen CB, Porsbjerg C, Astrup A, Bangsbo J, Parker D, Backer V (2018). Effects of exercise and diet in nonobese asthma patients—A randomized controlled trial. J Allergy Clin Imm Pract 6: 803-811.

Toennesen LL, Soerensen E, Hostrup M, Porsbjerg C, Bangsbo J, Backer V (2018). Feasibility of high-intensity training in asthma. Europ Clinic Resp J 5: 1468714.

Book

Bangsbo J. (2012). "Exercise and Training Physiology – A Simple Approach", pp. 1-190. SISU Sports Books, Sweden.